Lens AND Glaucoma

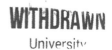

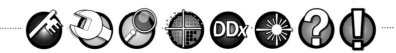

Rapid Diagnosis in Ophthalmology
Series Editors: Jay S. Duker MD, Marian S. Macsai MD
Associate Editor: Gary S. Schwartz MD

Anterior Segment
Bruno Machado Fontes, Marian S. Macsai
ISBN 978-0-323-04406-6

Lens and Glaucoma
Joel S. Schuman, Viki Christopoulos, Deepinder K. Dhaliwal,
Malik Y. Kahook, Robert J. Noecker
ISBN 978-0-323-04443-1

Neuro-ophthalmology
Jonathan D. Trobe
ISBN 978-0-323-04456-1

Oculoplastic and Reconstructive Surgery
Jeffrey A. Nerad, Keith D. Carter, Mark Alford
ISBN 978-0-323-05386-0

Pediatric Ophthalmology and Strabismus
Mitchell B. Strominger
ISBN 978-0-323-05168-2

Retina
Adam H. Rogers, Jay S. Duker
ISBN 978-0-323-04959-7

Commissioning Editor: Russell Gabbedy
Development Editor: Martin Mellor Publishing Services Ltd
Project Manager: Rory MacDonald
Design Manager: Stewart Larking
Illustration Manager: Merlyn Harvey
Illustrator: Jennifer Rose
Marketing Manager(s) (UK/USA): John Canelon/Lisa Damico

Series Editors: Jay S. **Duker** MD, Marian S. **Macsai** MD

Associate Editor: Gary S. **Schwartz** MD

Rapid Diagnosis in Ophthalmology
Lens AND
Glaucoma

By

Joel S. Schuman MD FACS, Professor and Chairman of Ophthalmology, University of Pittsburgh School of Medicine; Director, UPMC Eye Center; Professor of Bioengineering, University of Pittsburgh School of Engineering, Pittsburgh, PA, USA

Viki Christopoulos MD, Assistant Professor, Cornea and External Diseases/ Refractive Surgery, Department of Ophthalmology, University of Pittsburgh School of Medicine, UPMC Eye Center, Pittsburgh, PA, USA

Deepinder K. Dhaliwal MD, Associate Professor, Department of Ophthalmology, University of Pittsburgh School of Medicine; Director of Cornea and Refractive Surgery Services, UPMC Eye Center; Medical Director, Laser/ Aesthetic Center, University of Pittsburgh Medical Center, Pittsburgh, PA, USA

Malik Y. Kahook MD, Assistant Professor; Director of Clinical Research, Rocky Mountains Lions Eye Institute, University of Colorado at Denver and Health Sciences Center, Aurora, CO, USA

Robert J. Noecker MD MBA, Vice Chair, Clinical Affairs; Director, Glaucoma Service; Associate Professor, University of Pittsburgh School of Medicine, UPMC Eye Center, Eye and Ear Institute, Pittsburgh, PA, USA

Series Editors

Jay S. Duker MD, Director, New England Eye Center, Vitreoretinal Diseases and Surgery Service; Professor and Chair of Ophthalmology, Tufts University School of Medicine, Boston, MA, USA

Marian S. Macsai MD, Chief, Division of Ophthalmology, Evanston Northwestern Healthcare; Professor and Vice-Chair, Department of Ophthalmology, Feinberg School of Medicine, Northwestern University, Chicago, IL, USA

Associate Editor

Gary S. Schwartz MD, Adjunct Associate Professor, Department of Ophthalmology, University of Minnesota, Minneapolis, MN, USA

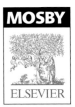

MOSBY

ELSEVIER

Mosby is an affiliate of Elsevier Inc.

© 2008, Elsevier Inc. All rights reserved.

First published 2008

ISBN 978-0-323-04443-1

British Library Cataloguing in Publication Data
A catalogue record for this book is available from the British Library

Library of Congress Cataloging in Publication Data
A catalog record for this book is available from the Library of Congress

Notice
Medical knowledge is constantly changing. Standard safety precautions must be followed, but as new research and clinical experience broaden our knowledge, changes in treatment and drug therapy may become necessary or appropriate. Readers are advised to check the most current product information provided by the manufacturer of each drug to be administered to verify the recommended dose, the method and duration of administration, and contraindications. It is the responsibility of the practitioner, relying on experience and knowledge of the patient, to determine dosages and the best treatment for each individual patient. Neither the Publisher nor the authors assume any liability for any injury and/or damage to persons or property arising from this publication.
The Publisher

your source for books,
journals and multimedia
in the health sciences

www.elsevierhealth.com

Working together to grow
libraries in developing countries

www.elsevier.com | www.bookaid.org | www.sabre.org

ELSEVIER   BOOK AID International   Sabre Foundation

The
publisher's
policy is to use
**paper manufactured
from sustainable forests**

Printed in China
Last digit is the print number: 9 8 7 6 5 4 3 2 1

Contents

5 Cataract

6 Open Angle Glaucoma

7 Closed Angle Glaucoma

Contents

8 Pediatric Glaucoma

Contents

Given the complexity and quantity of clinical knowledge required to correctly identify and treat ocular disease, a quick reference text with high quality color images represents an invaluable resource to the busy clinician. Despite the availability of extensive resources online to clinicians, accessing these resources can be time consuming and often requires filtering through unnecessary information. In the exam room, facing a patient with an unfamiliar presentation or complicated medical problem, this series will be an invaluable resource.

This handy pocket sized reference series puts the knowledge of world-renowned experts at your fingertips. The standardized format provides the key element of each disease entity as your first encounter. The additional information on the clinical presentation, ancillary testing, differential diagnosis and treatment, including the prognosis, allows the clinician to instantly diagnose and treat the most common diseases seen in a busy practice. Inclusion of classical clinical color photos provides additional assurance in securing an accurate diagnosis and initiating management.

Regardless of the area of the world in which the clinician practices, these handy references guides will provide the necessary resources to both diagnose and treat a wide variety of ophthalmic diseases in all ophthalmologic specialties. The clinician who does not have easy access to sub-specialists in Anterior Segment, Glaucoma, Pediatric Ophthalmology, Strabismus, Neuro-ophthalmology, Retina, Oculoplastic and Reconstructive Surgery, and Uveitis will find these texts provide an excellent substitute. World-wide recognized experts equip the clinician with the elements needed to accurately diagnose treat and manage these complicated diseases, with confidence aided by the excellent color photos and knowledge of the prognosis.

The field of knowledge continues to expand for both the clinician in training and in practice. As a result we find it a challenge to stay up to date in the diagnosis and management of every disease entity that we face in a busy clinical practice. This series is written by an international group of experts who provide a clear, structured format with excellent photos.

It is our hope that with the aid of these six volumes, the clinician will be better equipped to diagnose and treat the diseases that affect their patients, and improve their lives.

Marian S. Macsai and Jay S. Duker

Anomalies and abnormalities of the crystalline lens and the variety of the glaucomas can be simultaneously fascinating, complex and overwhelming. The sections that follow are designed to provide a rapid reference for a panoply of clinical entities, many of which present daily in physicians offices worldwide.

We have included quick facts for diagnosis and treatment, as well as photographs of the entities of interest. This section should be a ready reference for the busy clinician grappling with either familiar or unfamiliar findings. We hope that this information will be of benefit on both sides of the slit lamp.

Joel S. Schuman
Viki Christopoulos
Deepinder K. Dhaliwal
Malik Y. Kahook
Robert J. Noecker

We thank Diane Curtain for her tremendous photographic and artistic expertise, as well as her enthusiasm for education and her passion for our patients.

To our best teachers: our patients and our students.

To my mother Evelpia who is my angel and my children Constantine, Evely, and Thea who enchant me on a daily basis. VC

To my parents, Gurmeet and Amrik, and to my husband, Sanjiv, for their continued love and support. To my darling daughter, Diya, who is the light of my life. DKD

Acknowledgment/Dedications

Section 1
Congenital Abnormalities

Lenticonus and Lentiglobus

Key Facts

- Localized bulge (lenticonus) or generalized protrusion (lentiglobus) of anterior or posterior lens capsule
- Presumably due to lens capsular thinning
- Rare (1–4/100 000)
- Congenital or acquired
- Unilateral or bilateral
- Anterior rarer than posterior types
- Anterior lenticonus associated with Alport syndrome (90%)
- Posterior lenticonus usually idiopathic

Clinical Findings

- May present as progressive myopia, high astigmatism (irregular)
- Oil droplet reflex on retinoscopy
- Adjacent cortical opacification
- Uncommonly, spontaneous capsular rupture

Ancillary Testing

- None

Differential Diagnosis

- Galactosemia and galactokinase deficiency (oil droplet cataracts)
- Posterior polar cataract
- Persistent hyaloid remnants

Treatment

- **Cataract surgery if:**
  - associated lens opacity • high astigmatism • anisometropia

Prognosis

- Favorable on removal of associated cataract
- Vigilant postoperative occlusion to avoid amblyopia in children

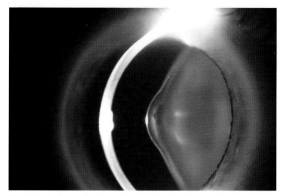

Fig. 1.1 A dramatic view of anterior lenticonus in a patient with idiopathic lenticonus.

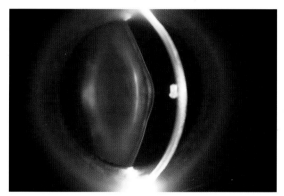

Fig. 1.2 The same patient also has posterior lenticonus. Although not as dramatic as his anterior lenticonus, the out-pouching of the posterior lens is still obvious.

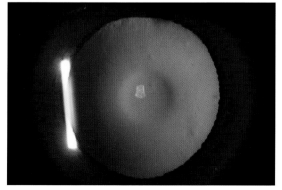

Fig. 1.3 The classic oil droplet reflex of lenticonus is best seen on retroillumination.

Lens Coloboma

Key Facts

- Equatorial lens flattening or notch due to a focal absence of lens zonules
- Underlying colobomatous ciliary body
- Usually sporadic (occasionally dominant)
- Unilateral or bilateral
- Isolated finding or associated with other ocular colobomas
- **Systemic associations:**
  - Patau syndrome (trisomy 13) • cat eye syndrome (trisomy 22) • coloboma, heart defects, choanal atresia, retarded development, genital and ear anomalies (CHARGE) • basal encephaloceles or cysts • Goldenhar syndrome • other syndromes

Clinical Findings

- Usually inferonasal quadrant
- Associated sectoral cataract
- Phacodonesis
- Often associated with colobomas of iris, ciliary body, retina, and choroid

Ancillary Testing

- None

Differential Diagnosis

- Lens-dislocating diseases (e.g. Marfan syndrome and homocystinuria)
- Adjacent pars plicata or ciliary body tumor (e.g. melanocytoma)
- Contusion or intraoperative trauma (acquired zonular defects)
- Normal variant (minor indentations between inserting zonules in young lenses)

Treatment

- Intervention usually not necessary
  - When cataract surgery is indicated, a capsular tension ring should be considered

Prognosis

- Excellent when isolated

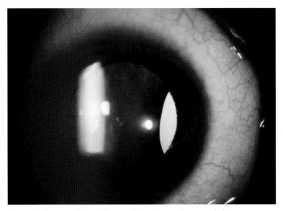

Fig. 1.4 A myopic patient with primary lens coloboma.

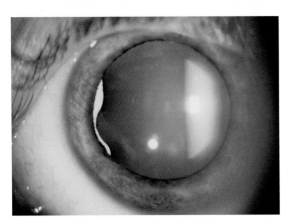

Fig. 1.5 Note the scalloped nasal edge of this 12-year old's lens coincident with absent lens zonules.

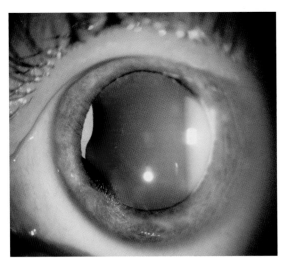

Fig. 1.6 Left eye of the same 12-year-old boy, taken at a different angle, showing a ciliary body cyst (seen inferonasally) as the cause of this secondary lens coloboma.

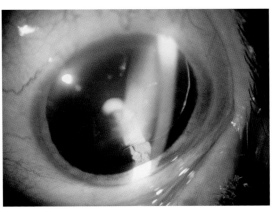

Fig. 1.7 Another case of secondary lens coloboma due to a ciliary body tumor.

Mittendorf Dot

Key Facts
- Remnant of the anterior end of the hyaloid vessel at posterior lens apex
- Sometimes associated with posterior lenticonus

Clinical Findings
- A grey-white dot opacity axial or nasal paraxial to lens posterior pole

Ancillary Testing
- None

Differential Diagnosis
- Posterior polar cataract
- Persistent hyperplastic primary vitreous
- Congenital cataract

Treatment
- Non-progressive, almost never requires surgery

Prognosis
- Visually insignificant

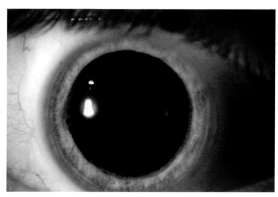

Fig. 1.8 A coincidental finding on routine eye examination, this Mittendorf dot was of no visual consequence (pictured here 180° away from the camera's light reflex). It is typically found just nasal to center.

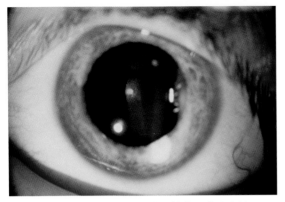

Fig. 1.9 A more dramatic example of Mittendorf dot in a 6-year-old girl (the persistent anterior hyaloid vasculature is shown in Fig. 1.10). The small posterior lens opacity, the once anterior hyaloid vessel attachment to the posterior lens capsule, is not an uncommon finding in routine eye examinations.

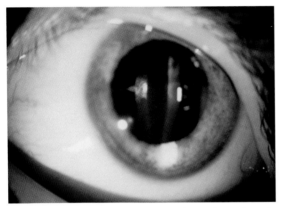

Fig. 1.10 The persistent anterior hyaloid vessel attachment at the posterior lens apex. A dramatic illustration of the anterior hyaloid vascular remnant attached to the posterior lens capsule.

Section 2
Developmental Defects

Marfan Syndrome

Key Facts

- Autosomal dominant (4–6/100 000)
- Mutation of fibrillin gene FBN1 on chromosome 15
- **Systemic features:**
  - tall • long limbs • arachnodactyly • flexible joints • pectus excavatum
    • high-arched palate • aortic dilation, valvular insufficiency, and dissection,
    and mitral valve prolapse

Clinical Findings

- Axial myopia, astigmatism
- **Lens:**
  - bilateral • superotemporal (two-thirds of cases) • lens subluxation (50–80%)
    or dislocation
- Zonules usually intact
- **Cornea:**
  - increased diameter • flatter
- Thin, blue sclera
- Glaucoma or angle anomaly
- **Iris:**
  - smooth, velvety appearance (lacks circumferential ridges, furrows, and crypts)
    • iridodonesis • transillumination (hypopigmentation of posterior iris pigment
    epithelium) • miotic (dilator muscle hypoplasia) • can be eccentric
- Cataract
- Lattice retinal degeneration, tears, and detachments

Ancillary Testing

- Keratometry (astigmatism mainly corneal)
- Biometry (long axial length measurements)
- Cardiac evaluation necessary
- Genetic counseling
- Work-up for aortic pathology

Differential Diagnosis

- Homocystinuria • Weill–Marchesani syndrome • Ehlers-Danlos
  syndrome • Sulfite oxidase deficiency • Hyperlysinemia • Congenital
  syphilis • Crouzon syndrome • Trauma • Ectopia lentis • Congenital
  glaucoma • Retinitis pigmentosa • Rieger syndrome • Medulloepithelioma

Treatment

- Initially, optimize refractive correction optically
- Consider optical iridectomy
- Lensectomy
  - Consider capsular tension rings, sulcus fixation, or sutured intraocular lenses

Prognosis

- Intraoperative complications can be high, although this is improving with newer
  endocapsular techniques
- Good surgical results can be limited by amblyopia

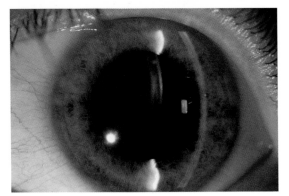

Fig. 2.1 Lenticular subluxation in a Marfan syndrome patient.

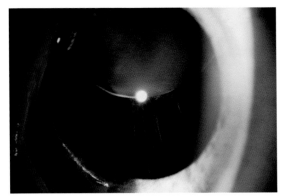

Fig. 2.2 Superior lens subluxation in a Marfan syndrome patient. The capsular lens zonules remain intact for the most part.

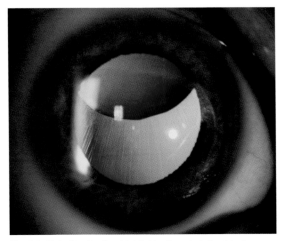

Fig. 2.3 Retroillumination highlights the stretched but mostly intact zonules.

Homocystinuria

Key Facts

- Autosomal recessive (1/200 000 in USA)
- Defect in cystathionine-β-synthetase
- Tall stature
- Mental retardation (50%)
- Coarse, fair hair
- Malar flush
- Skeletal abnormalities or osteoporosis
- Vascular thrombosis causes increased anesthesia risk via a yet unestablished platelet mechanism

Clinical Findings

- Progressive lenticular myopia or myopic astigmatism
- Blue irides
- Bilateral, inferonasal (57%) lens subluxation (90% incidence), lens dislocation
- Abnormal and broken zonules
- Possible pupillary block glaucoma
- Retinal vascular occlusions

Ancillary Testing

- Systemic work-up necessary
- Urine sodium nitroprusside spot test for homocystine for all children

Differential Diagnosis

- Hyperlysinemia
- Sulfate oxidase deficiency
- See differential diagnoses for Marfan syndrome (p. 10)

Treatment

- **Mild or severe subluxation:** optimize refractive correction
- **Moderate subluxation:** lensectomy may be necessary, because lens edge bisects pupillary axis
- Amblyopia therapy (patching in cases of anisometropia or strabismus)
- Consider Nd : YAG laser zonulysis to displace lens out of visual axis
- Consider laser pupilloplasty
- Consider optical iridectomy
- **Lensectomy:**
  - only if all other methods inappropriate • anesthetic thrombotic risk • bilateral lensectomy may be warranted to avoid second anesthetic risk • endocapsular tension rings intraoperatively
- **Systemic:** low methionine and high cysteine diet with supplemental pyridoxine (vitamin B_6) may prevent lens subluxation and mental retardation

Prognosis

- Intraoperative complications can be high, although this is improving with newer endocapsular techniques and perioperative measures to prevent thromboembolic events (diet therapy to increase cysteine and lower serum methionine and homocysteine levels, vitamin B_6 supplementation, good hydration, avoidance of hypoglycemia, perioperative antiplatelet drugs)
- Good surgical results can be limited by amblyopia

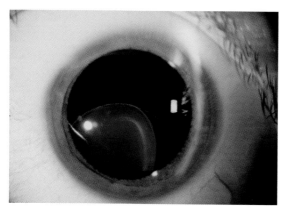

Fig. 2.4 Inferior displacement of the lens in a patient with homocystinuria.

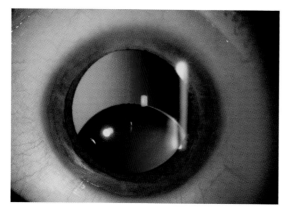

Fig. 2.5 Retroillumination of the same subluxed lens as in Fig. 2.4, highlighting the stretched, sometimes missing, zonules. The reduced zonular tension in this area tends to allow the equator edge to become thicker, thus increasing the patient's myopic prescription.

Ectopia Lentis

Key Facts

- Defined as displacement or malposition of the crystalline lens of the eye
- **Dislocated (luxed) lens:** the lens is in the anterior chamber or in the vitreous cavity
- **Subluxed lens:** the lens is displaced but contained within the normal lens space
- Caused by zonular laxity or disruption
- May be due to trauma (most common cause) or hereditary disorder
- Isolated ectopia lentis is autosomal dominant (chromosome 15)
- Ectopia lentis et pupillae involves displaced pupils in the opposite direction of lens subluxation and is autosomal recessive

Clinical Findings

- Poor vision
- Monocular diplopia
- Red painful eye when associated with trauma
- Abnormal red reflex or scissoring on retinoscopy
- Associated with Marfan syndrome, homocystinuria, Weill–Marchesani syndrome
- **Glaucoma occurs secondary to:**
    - lens dislocation in to the anterior chamber, resulting in pupillary block angle closure glaucoma • angle recession (after trauma) • associated angle dysgenesis

Ancillary Testing

- Dilated fundus examination
- B-scan ultrasonography (searching for dislocated lens)
- Retinoscopy shows myopia with astigmatism
- Appropriate systemic work-up when suspected

Differential Diagnosis

- Marfan syndrome (Fig. 2.1)
- Homocystinuria
- Weill–Marchesani syndrome
- Sulfite oxidase deficiency
- Hyperlysinemia
- Trauma (Fig. 2.2)

Treatment

- Laser peripheral iridectomy when pupillary block is present
- Pilocarpine once lens is posterior to iris, if lens is able to dislocate into anterior chamber
- **Lens extraction:**
    - often need pars plana approach if lens is luxed or significantly subluxed
    - capsular stabilizing devices are helpful when doing surgery on subluxed lens
    - sulcus or iris fixation of the intraocular lens is often indicated
- Topical hypotensive agents
- Evaluate and treat amblyopia

Prognosis

- Poor visual outcome if congenital with amblyopia
- Good prognosis with early detection or later manifestations

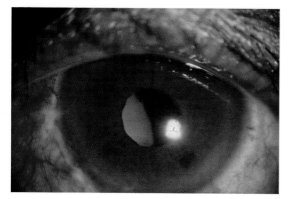

Fig. 2.6 Inferotemporal lens dislocation in a patient with Marfan syndrome.

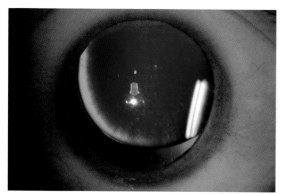

Fig. 2.7 Lens dislocation in a patient after blunt trauma.

Simple Ectopia Lentis

Key Facts

- Congenital or spontaneous non-traumatic displacement of the lens
- Usually autosomal dominant
- Bilateral, not always symmetric
- No systemic associations

Clinical Findings

- Myopia or astigmatism, frequently progressive during adulthood, can also present with diplopia and anisometropia
- Progressive lens displacement (usually superotemporal)
- Disrupted zonules
- Iridodonesis
- Cataract
- Glaucoma
- Retinal detachment
- Vitreous herniation

Ancillary Testing

- Retinoscopy
- Gonioscopy
- Work-up for aortic aneurysm (see Marfan syndrome, p. 10)

Differential Diagnosis

- Trauma (contusion or intraoperative) • Retinitis pigmentosa • Persistent pupillary membrane • Aniridia • Rieger syndrome • Megalocornea • Congenital syphilis • Homocystinuria • Weill–Marchesani syndrome • Ehlers–Danlos syndrome • Sulfite oxidase deficiency • Hyperlysinemia • Crouzon syndrome • Buphthalmos • Anterior uveal tumors • Marfan syndrome

Treatment

- **Mild ectopia:**
  - prescribe best optical correction
  - may tolerate rigid contact lenses better than spectacles, because of astigmatic correction
- **Advanced ectopia:** mydriatic therapy, aphakic correction (if lens displaced out of visual axis) or lensectomy (use of a capsular tension ring should be considered or sulcus fixation), or sutured intraocular lenses
- Options for rehabilitation after lensectomy include aphakic spectacles, contact lens correction, and intraocular lens implantation

Prognosis

- Significant visual impairment is unusual
- Amblyopia may lead to decrease in vision if not treated early

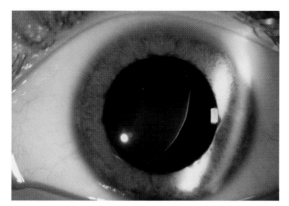

Fig. 2.8 Lens dislocation presenting as progressive myopia.

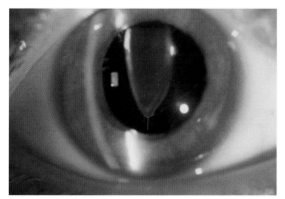

Fig. 2.9 The inferior zonules are maximally stretched in this 18-year-old's superiorly displaced ectopic lens.

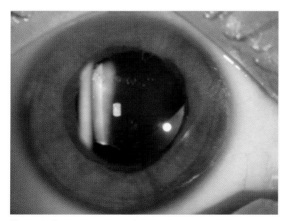

Fig. 2.10 Retroillumination of the same superiorly displaced ectopic lens as in Fig. 2.9.

Ectopia Lentis et Pupillae

Key Facts

- Congenital, non-traumatic displacement of lens and pupil
- <20% of ectopia lentis cases
- Autosomal recessive
- Bilateral, not always symmetric
- No systemic associations

Clinical Findings

- **Lens:**
  - myopia or astigmatism • progressive superotemporal lens displacement
    - disrupted zonules • microspherophakia • cataract
- **Iris:**
  - oval or slit pupil displaced in opposite direction of lens • iris transillumination
    - iridodonesis • pupil dilates poorly • persistent pupillary membrane
    - iridohyaloid adhesions • correctopia
- Glaucoma
- Retinal detachment

Ancillary Testing

- Ultrasound biomicroscopy (small pupil may not allow visualization)

Differential Diagnosis

- Same as for simple ectopia lentis

Treatment

- **Mild ectopia:** prescribe best optical correction, rigid contact lenses may be indicated
- **Advanced ectopia:** mydriatic therapy, aphakic correction (if lens displaced out of visual axis), or lensectomy
  - May require capsular tension ring, sulcus placement, or intraocular lens fixation
- Options for rehabilitation after lensectomy include aphakic spectacles (if bilateral), contact lens correction, and intraocular lens implantation

Prognosis

- Significant visual impairment is unusual

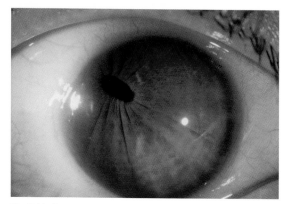

Fig. 2.11 A young adult with superotemporal pupil displacement (undilated).

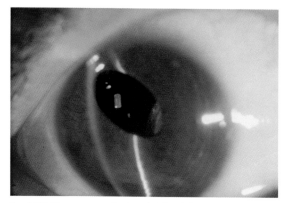

Fig. 2.12 The same patient as in Fig. 2.9 with pupil dilated, showing the inferonasal lens dislocation in the opposite direction to the pupil.

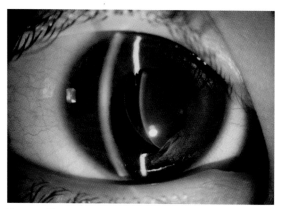

Fig. 2.13 The lens of this child is displaced superonasally in the opposite direction to the pupil. Compared with Figs 2.11 and 2.12, the pupil displacement is more subtle.

Weill–Marchesani Syndrome

Key Facts
- Autosomal recessive (high rate of consanguinity)
- Short stature
- Brachydactyly (short stubby fingers)
- Mental handicap uncommon

Clinical Findings
- Progressive myopia
- Microspherophakia
- Usually inferior or anterior lens subluxation
- Angle anomaly and pupillary block glaucoma

Ancillary Testing
- None

Differential Diagnosis
- Hyperlysinemia
- Sulfite oxidase deficiency
- See differential diagnoses for Marfan syndrome (p. 10)

Treatment
- Cycloplegic and mydriatic agents or iridectomy to relieve pupillary block
- Optical correction
- Lensectomy

Prognosis
- Variable

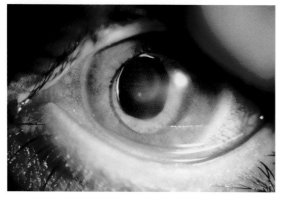

Fig. 2.14 Small lenses (microspherophakia) as in Weill–Marchesani syndrome. Spontaneous dislocation into the anterior chamber of a microspheric lens. (From Salmon J, Kanski J 2004 Glaucoma: a Colour Manual of Diagnosis and Treatment. Butterworth-Heinemann, Edinburgh.)

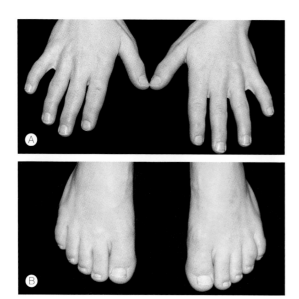

Fig. 2.15 Weil–Marchesani syndrome is inherited recessively and characterized by short stature and stubby fingers (A) and toes (B), which have stiff joints. Spherophakia, lenticular myopia of 10–20 D and lens dislocation are common. Heterozygotes may show a milder form of the disease. (From Spalton DJ, Hitchings RA, Hunter P 2005 Atlas of Clinical Ophthalmology, 3rd edn. Mosby, Edinburgh.)

Persistent Fetal Vasculature

Key Facts

- Unilateral abnormality associated with congenital cataract
- Persistence of the posterior fetal fibrovascular sheath of the lens
- Leukocoria

Clinical Findings

- Microphthalmos
- Shallow anterior chamber (lens thrust forward secondary to contracting retrolental membrane)
- Persistent pupillary membrane
- Cataract
- Ectopia lentis or ectopia lentis et pupillae
- Mittendorf dot
- Possible rupture of posterior lens capsule
- Retrolental, opaque membrane
- Elongated ciliary processes
- Iridohyaloid blood vessels
- Retinal folds or detachment

Ancillary Testing

- A- and B-scan ultrasonography
- CT scan or MRI (if poor posterior visualization and diagnosis and management cannot be determined by conventional techniques)

Differential Diagnosis

- Congenital cataract
- Retinoblastoma
- Toxocariasis
- Coats disease
- Persistent hyperplastic primary vitreous
- Retinopathy of prematurity
- Retinal astrocytoma
- Familial exudative vitreoretinopathy
- Uveitis
- Incontinentia pigmenti

Prognosis

- Visual prognosis poor, but early surgical intervention recommended to prevent phthisis and improve cosmesis
- Patient's visual function is normally good, because persistent fetal vasculature is unilateral

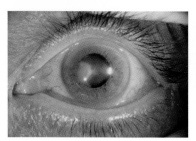

Fig. 2.16 Posterior subcapsular cataract with retrolental membrane in a patient with persistent fetal vasculature.

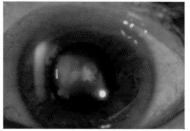

Fig. 2.17 A posterior subcapsular cataract as well as a nuclear cataract in the same patient as in Fig. 2.12.

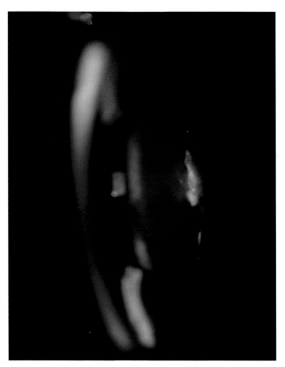

Fig. 2.18 Another view of the retrolental membrane: posterior subcapsular and nuclear cataract.

Section 3

Involutional Changes

Nuclear Sclerosis

Key Facts

- Opacification or sclerosis of the lens nucleus
- Blurring of distance vision greater than that of near vision
- Second sight myopic shift, can also see hyperopic shift with lens thickening
- May have monocular diplopia, glare loss of contrast, color vision changes
- Associated with prior pars plana vitrectomy

Clinical Findings

- Dense yellow or yellow-brown nucleus that is less translucent than surrounding cortex

Ancillary Testing

- Glare testing, potential acuity testing

Differential Diagnosis

- None

Treatment

- Lensectomy with intraocular lens implantation
- Spectacle or contact lens correction in the early stages

Prognosis

- Excellent following cataract extraction with intraocular lens implantation

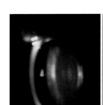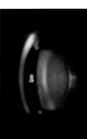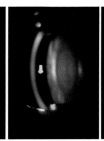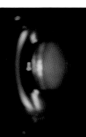

Fig. 3.1 Progressive yellowing of the lens (left to right) in nuclear sclerosis.

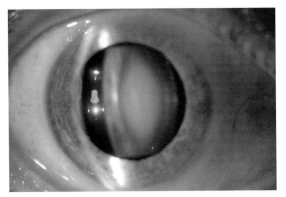

Fig. 3.2 Significant nuclear sclerosis.

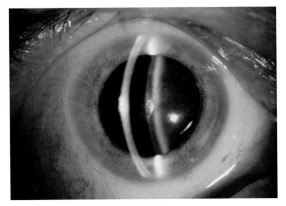

Fig. 3.3 A brunescent (literally "brown") lens.

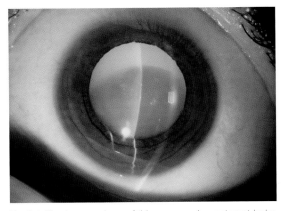

Fig. 3.4 The lens nucleus of this morgagnian cataract bobs freely within the capsular bag after complete cortical liquefaction.

Cortical Cataract

Key Facts
- Opacification of lens cortex
- Blurred vision, glare, and sometimes monocular diplopia may be visually insignificant

Clinical Findings
- **Stages:**
  - spoked cataract
  - white cataract (mature or complete cortical cataract)
- Hypermature cataract (leaky lens cortex produces anterior inflammation and glaucoma; phacolytic uveitis)
- Morgagnian cataract (complete cortical liquefaction allowing nucleus to move freely within the capsule)

Ancillary Testing
- Glare testing and potential acuity testing

Differential Diagnosis
- Hypocalcemia (small central white opacities)
- Fabry disease (cortical, spoke-like)
- Mannosidosis (cortical, spoke-like)
- Trauma, unknown etiology

Treatment
- Lensectomy with intraocular lens implantation when visually significant

Prognosis
- Excellent following cataract surgery

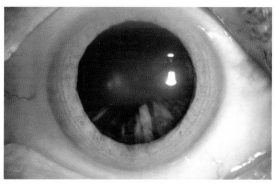

Fig. 3.5 Early inferior, sectoral cortical spokes, which are not yet symptomatic for this patient.

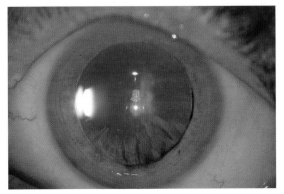

Fig. 3.6 Retroillumination of Fig. 3.5, highlighting the opacified inferior lenticular cortical spokes.

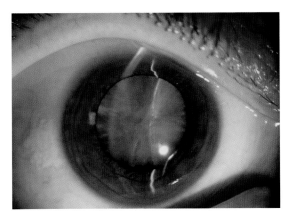

Fig. 3.7 A diabetic patient with a complete cortical cataract and underlying nuclear sclerosis.

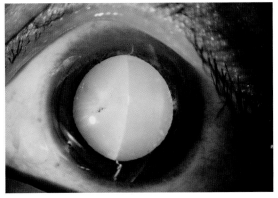

Fig. 3.8 A complete cortical cataract, often referred to as a white cataract.

Posterior Subcapsular Cataract

Key Facts

- Caused by posterior migration of equatorial lens epithelium, which causes focal or confluent opacification just beneath the posterior lens capsule
- Varied etiology (uveitis, corticosteroid use, diabetes, trauma, retinitis pigmentosa, prior intraocular surgery, trauma)
- Individual and ethnic characteristics may predispose to posterior subcapsular cataract (PSC; Hispanic people have a higher incidence of PSC than non-Hispanic people)
- Usually central

Clinical Findings

- Impaired near vision secondary to accommodative miosis
- Visually significant glare, worse under mesopic conditions
- Decreased contrast sensitivity (more than any other cataract type)
- **Specific morphologic PSC patterns can sometimes be seen:**
  - backbone of suture lines from which feathery opacities radiate (trauma) • focal and less opacified PSC (retinitis pigmentosa)

SECTION 3 • Involutional Changes

Ancillary Testing

- Near visual acuity testing with room lights on
- Glare testing
- Rule out systemic etiology, especially diabetes

Differential Diagnosis

- Congenital cataracts (plaque-like) • Myotonic dystrophy (plaque-like) • Turner syndrome • Fabry disease (sutural cataract) • Neurofibrosis type 2 • Posterior polar cataract • Mittendorf dot

Treatment

- PSCs may be rapidly progressive and require early surgical intervention
  - It is important during phacoemulsification to polish the posterior capsule, otherwise there is an increased risk postoperatively of posterior capsule opacification

Prognosis

- Excellent following cataract extraction with intraocular lens implantation

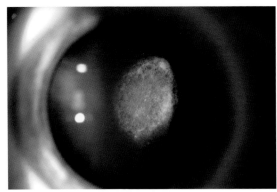

Fig. 3.9 This posterior subcapsular lens opacification has a lacy appearance. This patient reported a decrease in her visual acuity over 6 months, along with glare.

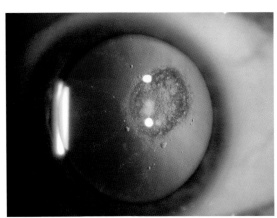

Fig. 3.10 View of the same posterior subcapsular cataract as in Fig. 3.9 with retroillumination.

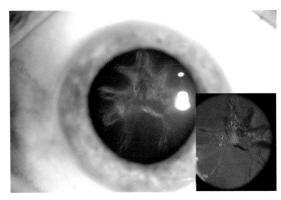

Fig. 3.11 A rather polypoidal appearance of the retroilluminated posterior subcapsular cataract shown in Fig. 3.10.

Polar Cataract

Key Facts

- Congenital plaque-like cataract located either anteriorly or posteriorly
- Posterior polar cataract is more common than the anterior polar type
- **Posterior polar cataract:**
  - a congenital form of cataract that extends anteriorly into the posterior cortex
    - usually autosomal dominant, sometimes sporadic • in many cases, there is a mutation in PITX3 gene, which is key in the role of lens and anterior segment development • sometimes associated with congenital defects in anterior segment development • can be associated with retinitis pigmentosa

Clinical Findings

- Symptoms of glare and visual complaints often out of proportion to degree of visual acuity
- Characteristic circular plaque-like opacity with concentric whorls
- With or without strabismus in a child
- With or without anterior segment dysgenesis
- Anterior polar cataracts may be associated with microphthalmos or microcornea
- Posterior polar cataracts may be associated with atopic keratoconjunctivitis

Ancillary Testing

- None other than detailed examination to include orthoptic testing and amblyopic prevention in children

Differential Diagnosis

- Anterior and posterior subcapsular cataracts
- Mittendorf dot
- Persistent hyperplastic primary vitreous

Treatment

- Cataract extraction if amblyogenic potential in children
  - It is necessary to perform a primary posterior capsulorrhexis in a young child
- Milder forms of posterior polar cataract that are discovered late in preschool children may require a trial of patching first to predict the timing of surgical intervention
- **In adults:**
  - posterior polar cataract should be removed only if very visually significant • surgical management of posterior polar cataracts can be challenging, in that it carries a high rate of posterior capsular rupture (up to 36% incidence) • there is a decreased incidence of posterior capsule rupture using a hydrodissection-free phacoemulsification technique (although this can make epinucleus removal more difficult), dissecting epinucleus peripherally first and centrally last, avoiding capsular polish and opting for YAG laser capsulotomy at a later date • slow-motion phacoemulsification using low settings or newer low-fluidic, low-vacuum bimanual phacoemulsification systems may decrease complications

Prognosis

- Usually good if uncomplicated surgery, although can be limited by amblyopia in unilateral or highly asymmetric cataract cases

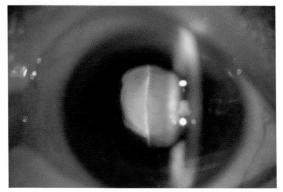

Fig. 3.12 A large, unilateral posterior polar cataract in a 70-year-old woman. She maintained excellent vision in her other eye and was able to easily accomplish her daily activities, therefore no surgical intervention was requested.

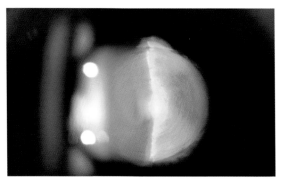

Fig. 3.13 A more magnified view of the same posterior polar cataract as in Fig. 3.12 shows its plaque- or disc-like quality. This cataract is much thicker than a posterior capsular cataract.

Section 4

Trauma

Perforation of Lens Capsule

Key Facts

- Cataract formation is the most common complication of penetrating ocular injury resulting in loss of vision
- Absorption of fluid between lens fibers (reversible), intracellular lens fiber swelling (irreversible)
- Surgical lensectomy is not always indicated

Clinical Findings

- Phacoanaphylactic (phacoantigenic) uveitis
- Increased IOP due to intraocular inflammation, peripheral anterior synechiae, papillary block, or angle recession
- Traumatic posterior rosette cataract (inflammatory cataract)

Ancillary Testing

- B scan
- CT scan to rule out the presence of an intraocular foreign body or open globe
- IOP monitoring

Differential Diagnosis

- Non-perforating blunt trauma (contusion rosette cataract)

Treatment

- First, thoroughly evaluate an open globe injury before management of lenticular injuries
- Medical management of inflammation and IOP
  - Surgical repair can be delayed if these are stable
- Miotics if monocular diplopia due to self-limiting, peripheral focal lens opacities
- **Lensectomy if:**
  - in conjunction with primary open globe repair
  - decrease in functional visual acuity
  - lens-induced inflammation or glaucoma
  - lens swelling from capsular rupture
  - poor visualization impeding management of posterior segment injuries

Prognosis

- Related to extent of injury and associated sequelae
- May lead to phacoantigenic uveitis or glaucoma if untreated

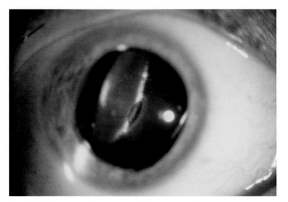

Fig. 4.1 Perforated lens capsule, caused by instrumentation during a vitrectomy, resulted in cataract formation within a few months. The lenticular trauma was not initially visible.

Intralenticular Foreign Body

Key Facts

- Minimal lens opacity and inflammation if the foreign body is completely embedded or encapsulated and if there is spontaneous capsule closure
- **Iron foreign body injury can lead to:**
  - direct siderosis (iron foreign body into lens)
  - siderosis bulbi (ionized iron in aqueous or vitreous)
  - chalcosis (>85% copper)
- Iron intraocular foreign bodies have more toxicity than alloy intraocular foreign bodies because they release more ions, which accumulate in lens epithelium
- Occult, small intraocular metallic foreign bodies are often the cause of more chronic manifestations of metallosis

Clinical Findings

- Heterochromia
- Mid-dilated, non-reactive pupil (pupillary sphincter muscle toxicity)
- Increased IOP
- Sectoral cataract surrounding foreign body
- Peripheral pigmentary retinal degeneration and sclerosed arterioles

Ancillary Testing

- CT scan or other imaging modality to evaluate extent of injury and to rule out additional intraocular foreign bodies
  - If metallic foreign body is suspected, a plain film x-ray can be used
- MRI should be avoided if metallic foreign body is suspected
- Electroretinogram (ERG) if posterior fundus findings (a decreased B-wave amplitude is a relatively sensitive finding in siderosis)
  - Serial ERGs are useful if surgical intervention is considered

Differential Diagnosis

- Lens iron pigmentation following an intraocular hemorrhage
- Wilson disease
- Congenital anterior polar cataract (pyramidal or with persistent pupillary membrane)

Treatment

- Intravenous antibiotics
- Lensectomy if vision compromised, metallosis, or endophthalmitis (7–30%)
- Intravitreal antibiotics many be necessary if early signs of endophthalmitis

Prognosis

- Variable depending on extent of injury
- Contaminated foreign bodies have a poor prognosis secondary to massive inflammatory response
- Deferring removal of larger intraocular foreign bodies for more than 24 h increases the risk of developing endophthalmitis from 3.5 to 13.4%

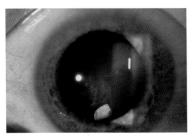

Fig. 4.2 A metallic foreign body lodged in the inferior lens and inciting cataractous changes.

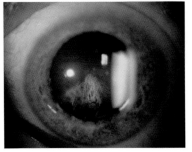

Fig. 4.3 Retroillumination of the eye shown in Fig. 4.2 highlights the localized inferior cortical cataract caused by the intralenticular iron foreign body.

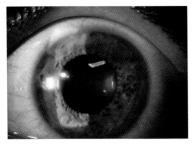

Fig. 4.4 A metallic foreign body lodged within the lens of a 30-year-old man (eye photographed at initial injury). The affected area soon became a cataract.

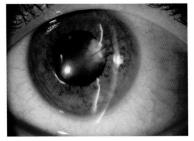

Fig. 4.5 Despite the removal of the metallic foreign body shown in Fig. 4.4, the patient developed a sectoral cataract most notable in the involved sector.

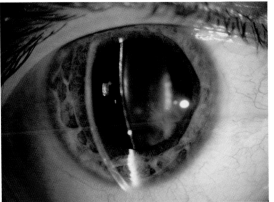

Fig. 4.6 Traumatic cataract resulting from a BB gun injury.

Radiation-induced Cataract

Key Facts

- The lens is the most radiosensitive ocular structure • Most susceptible if less than 1 year of age
- Radiation damages tumor DNA as well as cell membranes, causing germinative lens epithelial cells to swell, migrate posteriorly, and form posterior polar subcapsular cataract in 22–87% of eyes
- Stationary or progressive
- **Latency period:** months to years
- **Four stages:**
  1. posterior sutural opacities (caused by posterior migration of lens epithelial cells)
  2. a yellow-gold chromatic iridescence at the posterior pole (also caused by the extension of epithelium toward the posterior pole)
  3. stone-like opacities at the posterior pole
  4. immature cataract (secondary degeneration and liquefaction of posterior lens cortex)

Clinical Findings

- Posterior subcapsular cataracts more than anterior subcapsular cataracts
- Disc-like zone of opacification at equator and posterior pole
- Subcapsular vacuoles
- Liquefaction

Ancillary Testing

- Careful ocular examination to rule out radiation retinopathy, radiation keratitis, or optic neuropathy

Differential Diagnosis

- Posterior subcapsular cataract, diabetes

Treatment

- Lensectomy if visually significant
  - Because there is increased risk of posterior capsular disruption with advanced plaque-like posterior capsular cataracts, surgeons should err on the side of caution when performing hydrodissection
  - It is also important to polish the posterior capsule during phacoemulsification of mild posterior capsular cataracts to minimize the incidence of postoperative posterior capsular opacification
  - It may not be safe to polish the capsule of advanced posterior capsular cataracts, which sometimes necessitates YAG capsulotomy at a later date

Prognosis

- Dependent on retinal, tear function, and optic nerve status

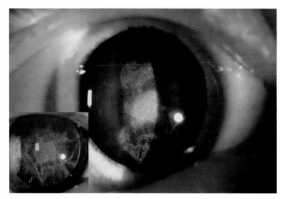

Fig. 4.7 Posterior subcapsular plaque after radiation therapy for cancer.

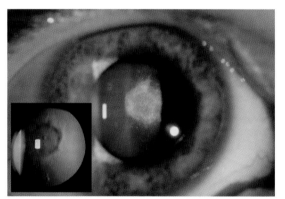

Fig. 4.8 A posterior subcapsular cataract affecting the central visual axis in another patient who had radiation therapy.

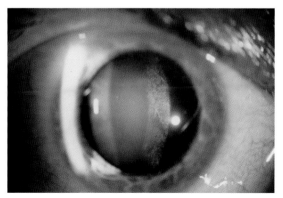

Fig. 4.9 A more diffuse subcapsular cataract in a 55-year-old man after radiation treatment.

Electric Shock Cataract

Key Facts

- Cataract is the most common change following electric shock
- Can occur after accidental electrocution, lightning strike, or electroconvulsive shock therapy
- High electric energy absorbed by the lens causes coagulation of lens proteins
- Melanin of the pigmented iris creates high resistance to electric currents, resulting in heat build-up, which further enhances cataract formation
- Occur 2–6 months after injury
- Amount of tissue destruction depends on voltage, amperage, resistance, pathway, and duration of current flow
- Lightning has anywhere from 20 million to 1 billion volts of electric energy and can occur by direct strike, side flash, spray, or ground strike

Clinical Findings

- **Acute:**
  - periorbital swelling or chemosis • ptosis • subconjunctival hemorrhage • thermal keratopathy • hyphema • uveitis • transient or permanent pupillary abnormalities (dilated or non-reactive pupils are unreliable indicator of severe brainstem hypoxia in cases of lightning) • vitreous hemorrhage • commotio retina • retinal detachment • central retinal vein occlusion • macular hole • chorioretinal rupture • thermal papillitis
- **Less acute:**
  cataracts
  - accommodation abnormality • lightning (anterior and posterior subcapsular cataracts with distinctive fern-like or starburst appearance) • industrial electric injury (anterior subcapsular cataract only) • dislocated lens
  posterior segment
  - lightning maculopathy (pigmentary changes) • retinal detachment • macular hole

Ancillary Testing

- B-scan ultrasonography if fundus not visualized

Differential Diagnosis

- Anterior and posterior subcapsular cataracts of another etiology

Treatment

- In an acute lightning strike, high-dose corticosteroids may be helpful in the presence of significant vision loss due to optic neuropathy
- Lensectomy

Prognosis

- Good if isolated cataract

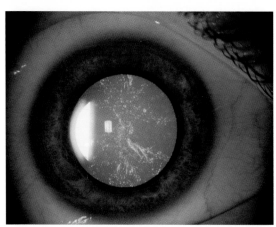

Fig. 4.10 Iridescent anterior and posterior lenticular changes forming a stellate pattern after a severe electric shock injury. The back of the patient's head fell on to a 6900-V wire.

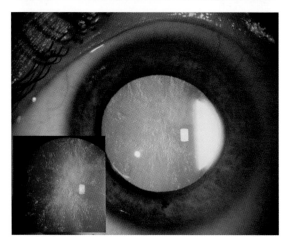

Fig. 4.11 A closer view of the other eye of the patient in Fig. 4.10, also with an electric shock cataract.

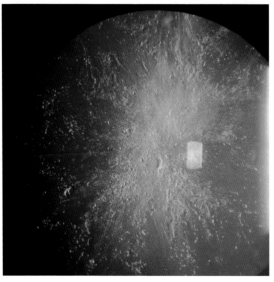

Fig. 4.12 A close-up of the eye shown in Fig. 4.11.

True Exfoliation (Glassblower's Cataract)

Key Facts

- Caused by thermal (infrared) injury, trauma, or intraocular inflammation
- First described in 1922 in glassblowers
  - Also found in steelworkers, blacksmiths, and workers in other occupations requiring direct exposure to intensely hot, open fires
- Lamellar splitting of the lens capsule, forming a scroll-like membrane on the lens surface

Clinical Findings

- Scrolls of lens capsule seen on dilation, with diaphanous membrane attached to the anterior lens capsule or rather inconspicuously in the anterior chamber

Ancillary Testing

- None

Differential Diagnosis

- Pseudoexfoliation syndrome

Treatment

- Lensectomy when visually significant
  - Capsulorrhexis can be more difficult in these patients, because the capsule can tear inconsistently
- Protective goggles imperative

Prognosis

- Good

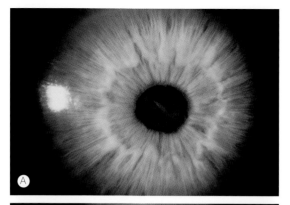

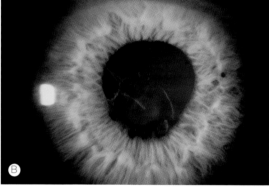

Fig. 4.13 Example of a true exfoliation cataract in a steelworker who had direct and intense infrared thermal exposure. During the boom of the steel industry, there were many cases of true exfoliation cataracts.

True Exfoliation (Glassblower's Cataract)

Section 5

Cataract

Inflammatory Cataract

Key Facts

- Secondary to chronic anterior or posterior uveitis
- The skin and lens share a common embryologic surface ectoderm origin, therefore the lens is affected in many dermatologic diseases and syndromes (e.g. atopic dermatitis)
- Corticosteroids, a major first-line treatment for inflammatory disease, can also cause cataract

Clinical Findings

- Blepharitis
- Conjunctival hyperemia and chemosis
- Keratoconus (e.g. atopy)
- Iritis
- Posterior synechiae
- Cataract
- Typically posterior subcapsular cataract
- Shield cataract (atopic dermatitis, anterior subcapsular cataract)

Ancillary Testing

- Optical coherence tomography to rule out macular edema

Differential Diagnosis

- Anterior and posterior subcapsular cataracts

Treatment

- **Lensectomy if visually significant:**
  - in children with active juvenile rheumatoid arthritis, no intraocular implant is placed
  - it is best to avoid anterior chamber intraocular lenses in uveitis patients

Prognosis

- Variable because of postoperative course (may develop persistent cystoid macular edema, epiretinal membrane, iritis, or inflammatory membrane over lens surface)
- Rate of posterior capsular opacification is higher than with other types of cataract

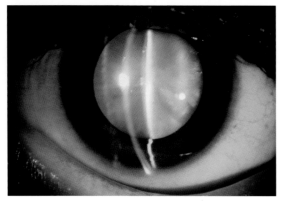

Fig. 5.1 A white cortical cataract secondary to atopic skin disease.

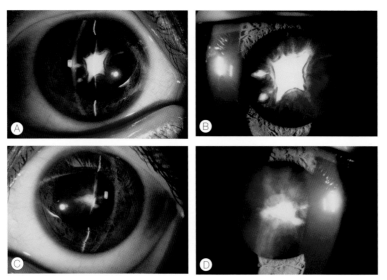

Fig. 5.2 (A) A shield-like anterior subcapsular cataract in another atopic patient with a history of longstanding topical steroid use. (B) Close-up of (A). (C) The patient's left eye also had a visually significant anterior subcapsular cataract. (D) Close-up of (C).

Inflammatory Cataract (Continued)

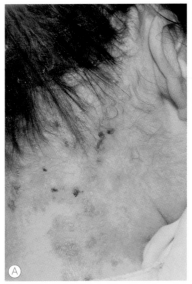
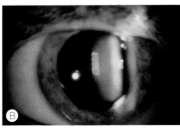

Fig. 5.3 (A) This 48-year-old woman treated her severe, longstanding dermatitis with chronic, intermittent use of topical steroid creams. (B) This plaque-like posterior subcapsular cataract developed as a result.

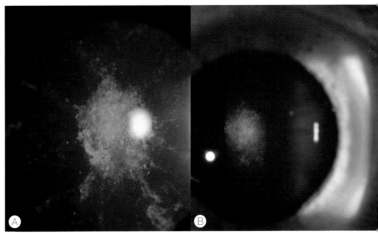

Fig. 5.4 (A) Magnified, retroilluminated image. (B) Posterior subcapsular cataract.

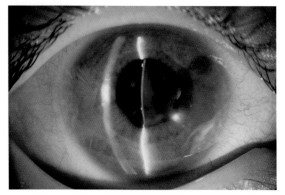

Fig. 5.5 A patient with recurrent acute anterior uveitis with posterior synechiae and a developing posterior subcapsular cataract.

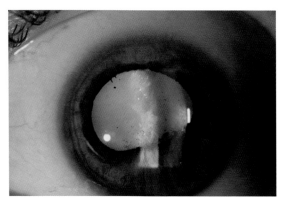

Fig. 5.6 Significant cortical cataract with inferior posterior synechiae in a 25-year-old woman.

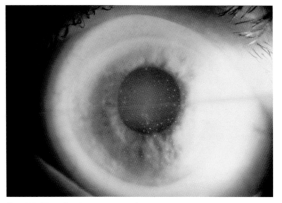

Fig. 5.7 Developing cataract in a patient with chronic, recurrent anterior uveitis and corneal keratitic precipitates.

Cataract Secondary to Diabetes

Key Facts

- Diabetes is one of the most important identifiable risk factors for cataract in western countries
- Elevated glucose within the lens causes metabolic conversion of excess glucose to sorbitol by the enzyme aldose reductase
- Increased lens sorbitol causes an osmotic shift drawing water into the lens, producing a reversible lens opacity and refractive shift
- Subsequent osmotic refractive changes can persist for up to 20 weeks after onset

Clinical Findings

- Transient and/or variable myopia, astigmatism, or hypermetropia (hyperglycemia or hypoglycemia)
- Cataracts
  Juvenile:
  - first three decades of life • subcapsular changes, cortical polychromatic opacities, vacuoles • reversible on treatment over time or progressive
  Adult:
  - posterior subcapsular more than nuclear, cortical • also polychromatic opacities and vacuoles • more quickly progressive

Ancillary Testing

- Rule out preoperative clinically significant macular edema (fundus fluorescein angiography to assess ischemia)
- OCT

Differential Diagnosis

- Nuclear, cortical, posterior subcapsular cataracts

Treatment

- Lensectomy with intraocular lens implantation (once diabetic retinopathy treatment completed)
- Use pre- and postoperative topical non-steroidals
- Consider intravitreal triamcinolone injection

Prognosis

- Favorable if no diabetic retinopathy or maculopathy present at time of cataract surgery
- Variable, depending on the grade and treatment history of the diabetic retinopathy present at time of surgery
  - There may be postoperative deterioration of diabetic retinopathy following cataract surgery, as a result of macular edema, retinal ischemia, and neovascularization
- Close observation of diabetic retinopathy following cataract surgery leads to earlier treatment and improved final visual outcome

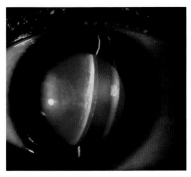

Fig. 5.8 Early-onset diabetic cataract developing in a 14-year-old African American girl with juvenile diabetes.

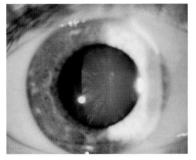

Fig. 5.9 Early cataractous changes in a 12-year-old with juvenile diabetes.

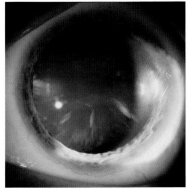

Fig. 5.10 Inferior cortical and early nuclear changes in an adult with non–insulin-dependent diabetes mellitus. He did not complain of any significant glare.

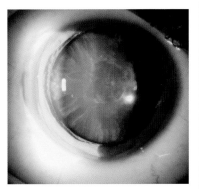

Fig. 5.11 Another variety of diabetic cataract. This patient had 20/200 (6/60) visual acuity.

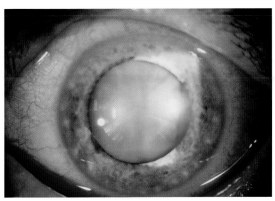

Fig. 5.12 This advanced cortical cataract appears white.

Myotonic Dystrophy (Christmas Tree Cataract)

Key Facts

- **Myotonic dystrophy:**
  - autosomal dominant (1/8000 incidence in white people)
  - a multiorgan disease (frontal alopecia, progressive muscular weakness, cardiomyopathy, abnormal smooth muscle motility, endocrinopathies, and infertility)
- Cataract may be only clinical feature of asymptomatic myotonic dystrophy
- Iridescent lens particles are subcapsular concentric inclusions (not crystals) of highly reflective, multilayered membranes
  - These inclusions appear polychromatic because of interference phenomenon

Clinical Findings

- Ptosis (orbicularis and levator muscle weakness)
- Oculomotor weakness
- Exphoria or exotropia
- Ocular hypotony
- Miosis or pupillary margin vascular tufts
- **Lens types:**
  - dusting of multicolored iridescent lens crystals in subcapsular cortical space
  - a stellate grouping of opacities along the posterior suture lines at the posterior pole
  - white cataract
- Rarely retinal pigmentary changes (abnormal electroretinogram responses)

Ancillary Testing

- Molecular testing now available for the diagnosis of myotonic dystrophy and identification of asymptomatic gene carriers (PCR used to specifically detect expansion of an unstable DNA sequence, CTG)
- Genetic counseling for younger generations of the family

Differential Diagnosis

- Cortical and subcapsular cataracts
- Juvenile diabetic cataract

Treatment

- Lensectomy if visually significant cataract

Prognosis

- Good
- Capsulorrhexis contracture and posterior capsular opacification reported (posterior capsule opacification can be recurrent)

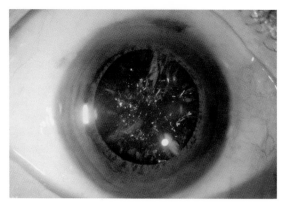
Fig. 5.13 Polychromatic lenticular changes are classically seen in patients with myotonic dystrophy.

Cataract Secondary to Ischemia

Key Facts

- Any cause of ischemia, including smoking-induced ischemia, increases the risk of cataract

Clinical Findings

- Lid edema
- Conjunctival chemosis
- Striate keratopathy
- Keratic precipitates
- Anterior chamber cell and flare
- Glaukomflecken (central, anterior subcapsular opacities secondary to acute angle closure glaucoma)
- Fixed pupil
- Iris neovascularization or atrophy
- Retinal hemorrhages, cotton wool spots, neovascularization
- Hypotony
- **Cataract:**
  - juvenile (white punctuate or snowflake posterior or anterior opacities)
  - adult (nuclear, cortical, or subcapsular opacities)

Ancillary Testing

- Carotid ultrasound in addition to cardiac referral

Differential Diagnosis

- Diabetes mellitus
- Radiation retinopathy (cataract with retinal hemorrhages)
- Uveitic (cataract with anterior chamber reaction)
- Galactosemia or galactokinase deficiency (oil droplet cataracts in infants)

Treatment

- Lensectomy with close postoperative follow-up

Prognosis

- Variable, depending on severity and cause of ischemia, retinal damage, iris disease, etc.

Section 6

Open Angle Glaucoma

Primary Open Angle Glaucoma

Key Facts

- Bilateral optic neuropathy
- May present initially as unilateral disease and progress at different rates between eyes
- Characteristic loss of retinal ganglion cells, optic nerve structural changes, and loss of visual function
- In 0.5–2% or more of population over 40
- Increased incidence with age
- Higher rate in persons of black African descent (three to six times)
- No sex predilection
- Asymptomatic until late stages

Mechanism

- Mechanism is poorly understood
- **Mechanical:** IOP too high for optic nerve, with resulting loss of retinal ganglion cells by apoptosis
- **Vascular:** poor blood flow to the optic nerve, resulting in hypoxia and apoptosis
- **Neurotoxicity:** apoptosis due to neurotoxins in neighborhood of retinal ganglion cells, cytokine activation, or reduction of growth factors

Clinical Findings

- **Always present:**
  - global and/or focal thinning of the retinal nerve fiber layer and optic nerve neuroretinal rim
- **Often present:**
  - cupping of the optic nerve, with a cup : disc ratio >0.3 (Fig. 6.1) • visual field defects respecting the horizontal meridian (i.e. nasal step, arcuate scotoma, paracentral defects; Fig. 6.2) • cup : disc asymmetry >0.2 • nasalization of blood vessels and focal thinning of vasculature at disc margin
- **Major risk factors:**
  - IOP > 21 mmHg • central corneal thickness <555 μm in the presence of elevated IOP • age (risk increases with increasing age) • family history of glaucoma • myopia • African American or Hispanic ancestry

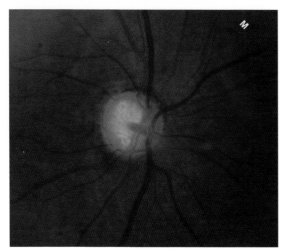

Fig. 6.1 Large cup : disc ratio with loss of neuroretinal rim.

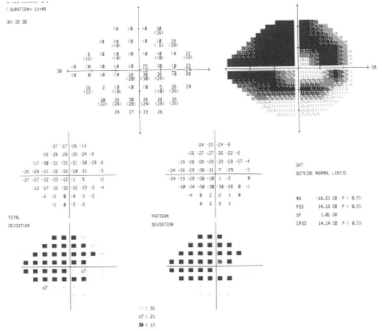

Fig. 6.2 Superior and inferior arcuate defects.

Ancillary Testing

- Gonioscopy
- Applanation tonometry
- Pachymetry
- Visual field
- Imaging (optical coherence tomography, GDx, Heidelberg retinal tomograph; Fig. 6.3)
- Stereoscopic optic nerve photographs are still the gold standard

Differential Diagnosis

- Ocular hypertension
- Physiologically large optic nerves or cups
- Secondary open angle glaucoma
- Chronic angle closure glaucoma
- Ischemic optic neuropathies
- Optic nerve coloboma
- Myopia
- Optic nerve pit

Treatment

- Ocular hypotensive drops
- Argon laser trabeculoplasty
- Selective laser trabeculoplasty
- Trabeculectomy
- Glaucoma drainage devices
- Endoscopic cyclophotocoagulation
- Trans-scleral cyclophotocoagulation

Prognosis

- Visual loss is permanent once it occurs
- Good prognosis with IOP control
- Worse prognosis in persons of African descent

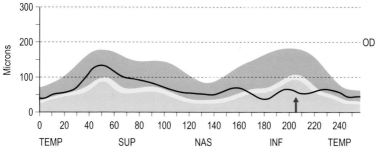

Fig. 6.3 Optical coherence tomogram of the retinal nerve fiber layer, showing thinning inferiorly.

Corticosteroid-related (Steroid Responders)

Key Facts

- Increased IOP is time- and dose-dependent
- 30% of population are steroid responders
- Up to 100% of primary open angle glaucoma (POAG) patients are steroid responders
- Occurs ≥2 weeks after starting topical corticosteroid therapy (sooner with oral and intravenous forms)
- May occur with various forms of corticosteroids (topical, inhaled, oral, etc.)
- IOP usually returns to presteroid use levels on withdrawal
- Chance that IOP will not return to presteroid levels is increased with longer corticosteroid usage

Mechanism

- **Increased resistance to outflow of aqueous at the level of the trabecular meshwork and Schlemm's canal due to one or more of the following:**
  - cytoskeletal changes • cytokine changes • myocilin abnormalities (synthesis, intracellular, extracellular) • abnormal extracellular protein deposition • endothelin-1 secretion by the non-pigmented ciliary epithelium
- Can be confusing in inflammatory glaucoma, in which aqueous production (generally reduced with inflammation) increases with steroid use, increasing IOP, but inflammation may decrease aqueous outflow with resultant increase in outflow and decrease in IOP with steroid treatment
  - Steroid response overlain on this clinical picture can be difficult to detect or tease out

Clinical Findings

- See *Primary open angle glaucoma* (p. 60)

Ancillary Testing

- See *Primary open angle glaucoma* (p. 60)

Differential Diagnosis

- See *Primary open angle glaucoma* (p. 60)
- Inflammatory glaucoma

Treatment

- Start ocular hypotensive agent if needed
- Withdraw steroids or decrease dose
- Use less potent forms of steroid (rimexolone, loteprednol, fluorometholone)
- See *Primary open angle glaucoma* (p. 60)

Prognosis

- IOP typically returns to presteroid levels with withdrawal
- May take months to return to baseline IOP
- Steroid responders are at higher risk to develop POAG in the future

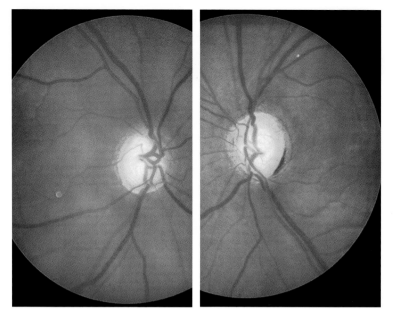

Fig. 6.4 Glaucomatous cupping, more advanced on the left than on the right, in a patient who had used topical steroids without supervision for treatment of mild ocular irritation associated with contact lens wear. (From Spalton DJ, Hitchings RA, Hunter P 2005 Atlas of Clinical Ophthalmology, 3rd edn. Mosby, Edinburgh.)

Inflammatory

Types

- Glaucoma secondary to uveitis
- Herpes simplex trabeculitis
- Herpes zoster ophthalmicus
- Syphilis
- Sarcoidosis

Key Facts

- Presents with pain, photophobia, and decreased vision
- May be asymptomatic
- Unilateral or bilateral
- Most cases idiopathic
- History of shingles or herpetic sores
- History of systemic diseases (ankylosing spondylitis, sarcoidosis, arthritis)
- Coexistent corneal findings (current or evidence of prior dendritic ulcers, pseudodendrites, band keratopathy)

Mechanism

- Outflow obstruction due to inflammatory cells
- Swelling of trabecular meshwork

Clinical Findings

- Inflammatory cells in anterior chamber
- Hyperemic conjunctiva
- Ciliary flush
- Peripheral synechiae (Fig. 6.5)
- Keratic precipitates on corneal endothelium
- Hypopyon (Fig. 6.6)
- Inflammatory cells in trabecular meshwork

Ancillary Testing

- See *Primary open angle glaucoma* (p. 68)
- Serology for systemic diseases associated with uveitis
  - erythrocyte sedimentation rate • angiotensin-converting enzyme • rapid plasma reagin • fluorescent treponemal antibody absorption • tuberculosis (purified protein derivative) • rheumatoid factor • antinuclear antibody • chest x-ray

Differential Diagnosis

- Steroid-induced (oral, intravenous, ophthalmic, dermal, or inhaled) • Chronic angle closure glaucoma • Primary open angle glaucoma

Treatment

- Ocular hypotensive drops • Cycloplegic drops • Steroid drops • Systemic immunosuppressives may be helpful in select cases • Treat underlying cause if any • Most often, no etiology is identified (idiopathic)

Prognosis

- Good prognosis if treated early
- May be recurrent with progressive damage

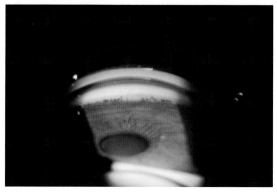

Fig. 6.5 Peripheral synechiae.

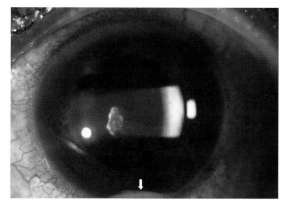

Fig. 6.6 Layering of inflammatory cells in the anterior chamber (hypopyon).

Normal Tension Glaucoma (Normal Pressure Glaucoma, Low-tension Glaucoma, Low-pressure Glaucoma)

Key Facts

- Progressive optic neuropathy similar to primary open angle glaucoma (POAG)
- No documented IOP > 22 mmHg
- Higher rate of disc hemorrhages than in POAG
- Visual field defects may be more likely to be dense and paracentral
- High association with migraine and autoimmune disease
- IOP still a causal factor in optic neuropathy despite statistically normal level

Mechanism

- Pressure-dependent and pressure-independent factors
- IOP
- Ocular blood flow
- Neurotoxicity
- **Possible etiologies:**
  - poor structural support of nerve at lamina cribrosa • autoimmune disease • hypotensive episodes • vasospasm

Clinical Findings

- Optic nerve head cupping and cup : disc asymmetry
- Retinal nerve fiber layer defects (Fig. 6.7)
- Disc hemorrhages (Fig. 6.8)
- Normal IOP
- Similar to POAG
- Open angle on gonioscopy
- Association with migraine, Raynaud syndrome

Ancillary Testing

- See *Primary open angle glaucoma* (p. 60)
- Consider autoimmune work-up if history dictates
- **Consider MRI or CT of head and orbits to rule out intracranial etiology if:**
  - patient younger than 50 • visual fields do not match optic nerve examination • rapidly progressive visual field changes • optic nerve head pallor • unilateral process • localizing neurologic defects

Differential Diagnosis

- POAG
- Ischemic optic neuropathies
- Steroid-induced glaucoma
- Intermittent angle closure glaucoma
- Optic neuritis
- Trauma

Treatment

- See *Primary open angle glaucoma* (p. 60)

Prognosis

- Worse prognosis than for POAG

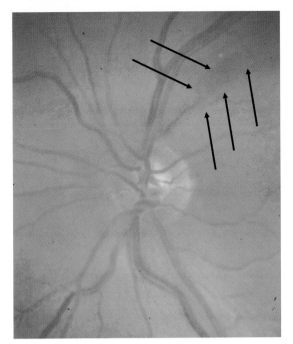

Fig. 6.7 Retinal nerve fiber layer defect outlined by arrows.

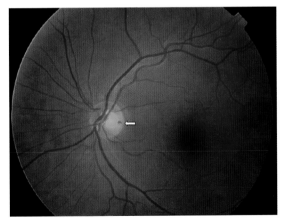

Fig. 6.8 Disc hemorrhage (arrow).

Pseudoexfoliation

Key Facts

- Most common identifiable cause of open angle glaucoma
- Exact etiology unknown
- Systemic disease
- May be a basement membrane disease (aggregates resemble amyloid)
- More common in older age groups (60–70 years of age)
- Bilateral (often asymmetric), rarely unilateral
- 40–60% of pseudoexfoliation (PXF) syndrome patients develop ocular hypertension or glaucoma
- Increased diurnal fluctuations compared with primary open angle glaucoma (POAG)
- Cataract surgery potentially more complicated in PXF secondary to poor pupillary dilation, a more fragile capsular bag, and weakened zonules

Mechanism

- Unknown etiology of PXF material formation
- IOP rise linked to trabecular cell dysfunction and blockage of drainage angle

Clinical Findings

- PXF material on lens capsule and iris
- Bull's-eye appearance to anterior lens capsule PXF material (Fig. 6.9)
- Uneven salt and pepper pigmentation of the angle (Fig. 6.10)
- Peripupillary iris atrophy or loss of pupillary ruff (Fig. 6.11)
- Phacodonesis
- Lens subluxation
- Sampaolesi's line (pigmented line anterior to Schwalbe's line)
- Endothelial cells are decreased with guttae formation
- Occasionally PXF material on corneal endothelium and iris

Ancillary Testing

- Similar to that for POAG

Differential Diagnosis

- POAG
- Pigmentary glaucoma
- Capsular delamination (true exfoliation)
- Primary amyloidosis

Treatment

- See *Primary open angle glaucoma* (p. 60)
- PXF glaucoma tends to respond to argon laser trabeculoplasty and selective laser trabeculoplasty but for a shorter duration compared with POAG, with sudden rapid failure

Prognosis

- Not all PXF patients progress to glaucoma
- Patients tend to do worse than those with POAG once glaucoma develops

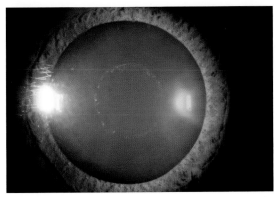

Fig. 6.9 Pseudoexfoliation material on anterior lens capsule with bull's-eye formation.

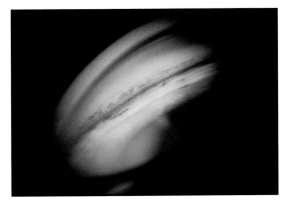

Fig. 6.10 Gonioscopic view showing coarse pigmentation of drainage angle.

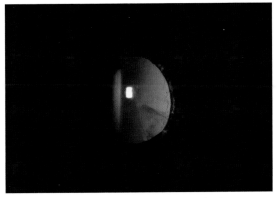

Fig. 6.11 Pupillary ruff atrophy with transillumination defects.

Pigmentary Glaucoma

Key Facts

- Results from effects of iris pigment toxicity to trabecular meshwork
- Pigment released from posterior iris surface because of midperipheral iridozonular contact
- More common in myopic young men
- Begins in third decade and severity decreases with time
- May be more common in white patients
- IOP may increase with exercise

Mechanism

- Midperipheral iridozonular contact with release of pigment from iris into aqueous humor
- Reverse pupillary block with lens–iris ball valve effect with blinking likely cause of iris concavity and iridozonular contact
- Released pigment causes trabecular endothelial cell dysfunction

Clinical Findings

- Krukenberg's spindle on corneal endothelium (Fig. 6.12)
- Trabecular meshwork velvety, homogeneous pigmentation (Fig. 6.13)
- Midperipheral transillumination defects in a radial spoke-like distribution (Fig. 6.14)
- Pain, haloes, decreased vision after exercise or dilation
- Higher rate of lattice degeneration (myopia)

Ancillary Testing

- See *Primary open angle glaucoma* (p. 60)
- Ultrasound biomicroscopy or gonioscopy shows an open angle, deep anterior chamber, and concave peripheral iris

Differential Diagnosis

- Primary open angle glaucoma (POAG)
- Pseudoexfoliation syndrome
- Inflammatory glaucoma

Treatment

- See *Primary open angle glaucoma* (p. 60)
- Generally responds well to laser trabeculoplasty but for shorter periods than POAG
- Miotic drops change iris contour and decrease iridozonular contact (induced relative pupillary block)
- Laser peripheral iridectomy changes iris contour and decreases iridozonular contact

Prognosis

- 35% of patients with pigment dispersion syndrome develop glaucoma over long term
- Pigmentary glaucoma most often develops within 15 years of pigment dispersion diagnosis
- Male sex, high myopia, and Krukenberg's spindles may portend a worse prognosis
- It is the one type of glaucoma that becomes easier to treat over time

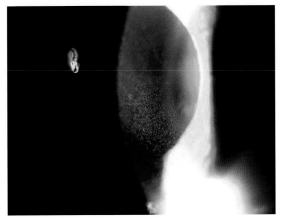

Fig. 6.12 Krukenberg's spindle showing pigment on corneal endothelium.

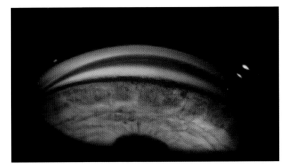

Fig. 6.13 Gonioscopic view showing heavy uniform pigmentation of drainage angle.

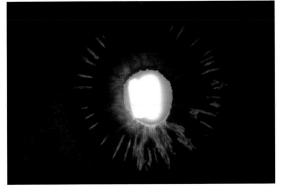

Fig. 6.14 Midperipheral transillumination defects in a radial spoke-like distribution.

Lens-induced: Phacolytic (Lens Protein)

Key Facts

- Several glaucomas can present with formation of cataracts
- The lens-induced glaucomas involving an open angle present with similar clinical signs and symptoms—careful examination and history taking are necessary to make the proper diagnosis and guide treatment

Mechanism

- **Phacolytic:** obstruction of trabecular meshwork by high molecular weight lens proteins leaking out of a hypermature lens
  - Macrophages are conspicuously present

Clinical Findings

- **Common findings:**
  - decreased vision
  - pain
  - photophobia
  - corneal edema
  - ciliary injection or red eye
- **Specific findings:**
  - hypermature cataract with wrinkles and/or plaques on anterior lens capsule (Fig. 6.15)
  - macrophage aggregates on anterior lens capsule
  - heavy flare with slow-moving particles in anterior chamber

Ancillary Testing

- B scan in cases of hypermature cataract to examine posterior structures

Differential Diagnosis

- Inflammatory glaucoma
- Endophthalmitis after surgery or trauma
- Acute angle closure glaucoma

Treatment

- Same as for primary open angle glaucoma for pressure
- Topical steroids to control inflammation
- Removal of lens and/or lens material for definitive treatment

Prognosis

- Excellent prognosis if definitive treatment is taken early with pressure control

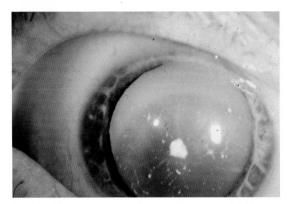

Fig. 6.15 Hypermature lens (morgagnian cataract) with nucleus sinking to the bottom.

Lens-induced: Lens Particle

Key Facts

- The lens-induced glaucomas involving an open angle present with similar clinical signs and symptoms—careful examination and history taking are necessary to make the proper diagnosis and guide treatment

Mechanism

- **Lens particle:** inflammatory reaction to exposed lens material after trauma or surgery, causing obstruction of trabecular meshwork outflow

Clinical Findings

- **Common findings:**
  - decreased vision
  - pain
  - photophobia
  - corneal edema
  - ciliary injection or red eye
- **Specific findings:**
  - heavy anterior chamber inflammation in a postsurgical or post-traumatic eye
  - fluffy lens material in anterior chamber

Ancillary Testing

- Gonioscopy to check for retained lens material in angle

Differential Diagnosis

- Inflammatory glaucoma
- Endophthalmitis after surgery or trauma
- Acute angle closure glaucoma

Treatment

- Same as for primary open angle glaucoma for pressure
- Topical steroids to control inflammation
- Removal of lens and/or lens material for definitive treatment

Prognosis

- Excellent prognosis if definitive treatment is taken early with pressure control

Lens-induced: Phacoantigenic

Key Facts
- The lens-induced glaucomas involving an open angle present with similar clinical signs and symptoms—careful examination and history taking are necessary to make the proper diagnosis and guide treatment

Mechanism
- **Phacoantigenic (also called phacoanaphylactic):** zonal granulomatous response after immunologic sensitization to exposed lens proteins after trauma or surgery

Clinical Findings
- **Common findings:**
  - decreased vision
  - pain (milder than in other forms of lens-induced glaucoma)
  - photophobia (mild)
  - corneal edema
  - ciliary injection or red eye
- **Specific finding:**
  - mild to moderate anterior chamber inflammation in postsurgical or post-traumatic eye after latent period

Ancillary Testing
- Gonioscopy to check for retained lens material in angle

Differential Diagnosis
- Inflammatory glaucoma
- Endophthalmitis after surgery or trauma
- Acute angle closure glaucoma

Treatment
- Same as for primary open angle glaucoma for pressure
- Topical steroids to control inflammation
- Removal of lens and/or lens material if present for definitive treatment

Prognosis
- Excellent prognosis if definitive treatment is taken early with pressure control
- Glaucoma is an infrequent complication of phacoanaphylaxis

Posner–Schlossmann Syndrome (Glaucomatocyclitic Crisis)

Key Facts

- Unilateral
- Young to middle-aged patients
- Very mild recurrent anterior chamber cellular reaction in otherwise quiet eye
- Self-limited episodes with quiet intervals
- Associated with HLA-Bw54

Mechanism

- Unknown

Clinical Findings

- Very high IOP (40–60 mmHg)
- Few fine keratic precipitates (Fig. 6.16)
- May have mid-dilated pupil
- Corneal edema
- Conjunctiva usually unaffected, rarely mildly hyperemic (Fig. 6.17)
- Lid edema, decreased vision, pain, nausea, and one-sided headache

Ancillary Testing

- See *Primary open angle glaucoma* (p. 60)
- Serology to rule out systemic causes of uveitis if recurrent

Differential Diagnosis

- Idiopathic uveitis
- Lens-induced uveitis
- Infectious uveitis
- Fuchs heterochromic iridocyclitis

Treatment

- Ocular hypotensive drops
- Topical steroids are of questionable benefit because individual episodes resolve spontaneously, regardless of treatment

Prognosis

- Good prognosis, with no treatment needed between episodes

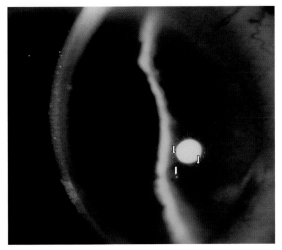

Fig. 6.16 Fine keratic precipitates (arrows).

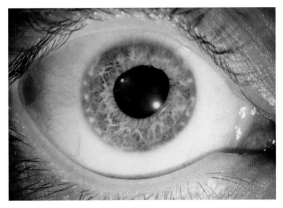

Fig. 6.17 Absent conjunctival hyperemia in a patient with Posner–Schlossmann syndrome.

Fuchs Heterochromic Iridocyclitis

Key Facts

- Unilateral iritis (90%)
- Age 30–40
- No sex predilection
- Usually asymptomatic until cataract development affects vision
- Higher rate in patients with light-colored irides

Mechanism

- Unknown
- May be related to depression of suppressor T cells

Clinical Findings

- Heterochromia (lighter colored iris on side of disease, rarely darker iris on side of disease; Fig. 6.18)
- Diffuse stellate keratic precipitates (Fig. 6.19)
- Mild anterior chamber cell reaction
- Cataract (70%)
- Minimal, if any, conjunctival hyperemia
- Fine fragile neovascularization of iris and angle in chronic disease
- Absent peripheral synechiae

Ancillary Testing

- See *Primary open angle glaucoma* (p. 60)
- Serology to rule out systemic causes of uveitis (usually not necessary)

Differential Diagnosis

- Idiopathic uveitis
- Infectious uveitis
- Posner–Schlossmann syndrome
- Tumor
- Steroid response

Treatment

- Topical hypotensive drops
- Unresponsive to steroids

Prognosis

- Reported rates of glaucoma vary between 13 and 59%
- When present, glaucoma often difficult to manage with medical therapy
- Surgical outcomes fair

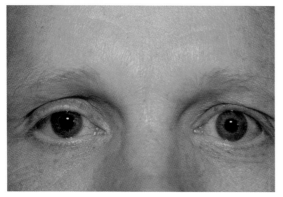

Fig. 6.18 Heterochromia.

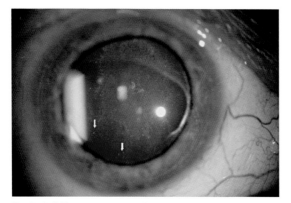

Fig. 6.19 Diffuse stellate keratic precipitates (white arrows).

Tumor-related Glaucoma

Key Facts

- Elevated IOP in 5% of all eyes with intraocular tumors
- Anterior uveal tumors lead to increased IOP in 41–45% of involved eyes
- Posterior uveal tumors lead to increased IOP in 14%
- Ring melanoma (involving 360° of ciliary body) leads to elevated IOP in 100% of involved eyes
- Intraocular tumors cause increased IOP through several mechanisms (see below)
- Intraocular tumors may cause open angle glaucoma through seeding of cells and direct expansion into angle
- Alternatively, tumors may cause closed angle glaucoma through direct mechanical closure of angle with anterior iris or lens displacement

Mechanism

- Direct tumor invasion of the angle (e.g. iris or ciliary body melanoma)
- Hemorrhage with migration of red blood cells into the angle
- Ghost cell glaucoma
- Tumor cells obstructing angle (leukemia, lymphoma)
- Inflammatory process with synechiae formation

Clinical Findings

- Often asymptomatic
- Decreased vision
- Increased IOP
- Pain
- Systemic symptoms depending on etiology
- Mass involving ciliary body and drainage angle (Figs 6.20 and 6.21)

Ancillary Testing

- B-scan or high-resolution anterior chamber ultrasound
- Ultrasound biomicroscopy
- Fluorescein angiography
- Gonioscopy
- Anterior or posterior chamber fine needle cell aspiration for cytology
- Systemic work-up for metastasis if indicated

Differential Diagnosis

- Primary open angle glaucoma
- Inflammatory glaucoma
- Hyphema
- Malignant glaucoma

Treatment

- Treat IOP elevation
- Cycloplegia
- Radiation, chemotherapy, or surgical excision of tumor as necessary

Prognosis

- Poor

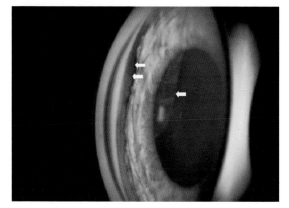

Fig. 6.20 Ciliary body melanoma visible through the pupil.

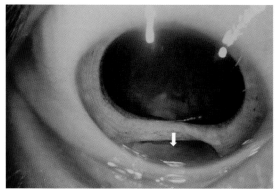

Fig. 6.21 Large ciliary body mass extending into the angle and anterior to the iris.

Elevated Episcleral Pressure

Possible Causes

- Carotid cavernous fistula
- Dural sinus fistula
- Graves orbitopathy
- Idiopathic
- Orbital varix
- Sturge–Weber syndrome
- Superior vena cava syndrome
- Retrobulbar tumor

Key Facts

- Uncommon form of glaucoma
- Unilateral (more common) or bilateral
- Diagnosing cause of increased episcleral pressure is key

Mechanism

- High IOP due to increased outflow resistance with higher than average episcleral vein pressure
- (Population average episcleral venous pressure is 8–10 mmHg)

Clinical Findings

- Blood visible in Schlemm's canal on gonioscopy (Fig. 6.22)
- Dilated and/or tortuous episcleral vessels (Fig. 6.23)
- Glaucomatous optic nerve changes
- Occasionally low-grade anterior chamber flare or cell

Ancillary Testing

- **Gonioscopy:** blood in Schlemm's canal is key finding
- See *Primary open angle glaucoma* (p. 60)
- Thyroid studies
- Orbital imaging (B scan, CT, MRI)
- Angiography or magnetic resonance angiography

Differential Diagnosis

- Primary open angle glaucoma
- Conjunctivitis
- Episcleritis
- Inflammatory glaucoma

Treatment

- Treat underlying cause, if known
- Increased chance of suprachoroidal hemorrhage with incisional surgery
- Responds better to topical therapy targeting aqueous production than topical therapy targeting outflow facility

Prognosis

- Good prognosis if discovered early

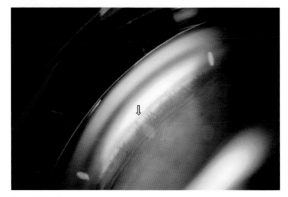

Fig. 6.22 Blood in Schlemm's canal (yellow arrow).

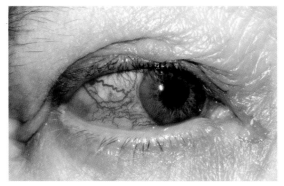

Fig. 6.23 Dilated episcleral vessels.

Sturge–Weber Syndrome (Encephalotrigeminal Angiomatosis)

Key Facts

- Incidence is 1 in 50 000 in the USA
- No race or sex predilection
- Angiomas of the leptomeninges and facial skin (V1 and V2 distribution)
- Port wine stain angioma of facial skin
- Seizures and developmental delay may occur
- Angioma represents failure of embryonal vessel regression
- Between 30–70% of Sturge–Weber patients have glaucoma
- About two thirds of those who have glaucoma will develop signs by 24 months of age

Mechanism

- Increased episcleral venous pressure leads to increased IOP and optic nerve damage

Clinical Findings

- Elevated IOP
- Facial hemangioma (Fig. 6.24), usually respecting midline
- Hemangioma affecting the upper eyelid is more frequently associated with elevated IOP
- Choroidal hemangioma in 40%
- Conjunctival or episcleral hemangiomas (Fig. 6.25)
- Large corneal diameter
- Photophobia
- Epiphora
- Blepharospasm
- Buphthalmos

Ancillary Testing

- Dilated fundus examination to check for choroidal hemangiomas
- Gonioscopy may show blood in Schlemm's canal
- Skull x-ray shows classic railroad track calcifications
- Electroencephalogram to evaluate for seizures

Differential Diagnosis

- None

Treatment

- Topical hypotensive agents
- Cyclodestructive procedures
- Trabeculectomy and glaucoma drainage procedures often needed
- High risk of suprachoroidal hemorrhage with penetrating surgery
- Use of an anterior chamber maintainer and prophylactic sclerotomies during glaucoma surgery may decrease rate of suprachoroidal hemorrhage

Prognosis

- Can be difficult to manage
- Frequently fails medical management
- Trabeculotomy or goniotomy in younger patients (effective in 66% with 5-year follow-up)
- Trabeculectomy and glaucoma drainage devices
- Ahmed valves have a 30% success rate after 60 months

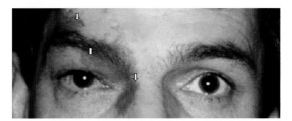

Fig. 6.24 Facial hemangioma (arrows) respecting midline.

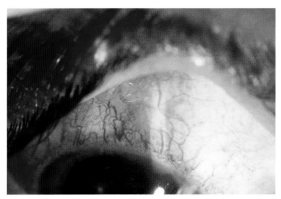

Fig. 6.25 Prominent episcleral vessels.

Traumatic

- Hyphema • Trabecular tear or trabeculitis • Angle recession • Iridodialysis • Cyclodialysis • Lens dislocation • Retinal dialysis or retinal tear • Ghost cell glaucoma

Key Facts

- Approximately 1 million ocular injuries occur each year • Most frequently affects young men • Boxing and contact sports are frequent causes • Glaucoma may manifest years after traumatic occurrence • Often unilateral • Increased risk of future glaucoma if hyphema present • Angle recession occurs in 60–94% of eyes after hyphema • 4–9% of patients with 180° angle recession develop glaucoma

Mechanism

- **Hyphema:** blood layering in anterior chamber (Fig. 6.26)
- **Angle recession:** tear between the longitudinal and circular muscles of the ciliary body (Fig. 6.27)
- **Iridodialysis:** a tear in the root of the iris (Fig. 6.28)
- **Cyclodialysis:** separation of the ciliary body from the scleral spur
- **Ghost cell:** degenerated blood cells block trabecular meshwork
- **Hemolytic glaucoma:** macrophages obstruct trabecular meshwork after ingesting red blood cells

Clinical Findings

- Decreased vision • Pain • Photophobia • Redness • Periorbital edema • Cataract • Vitreous hemorrhage • Pigment clumps on trabecular meshwork is a late sign of hyphema • Widening of ciliary body band is a sign of angle recession

Ancillary Testing

- Ultrasound biomicroscopy • B-scan ultrasonography • Gonioscopy • Head CT or x-ray • See *Primary open angle glaucoma* (p. 68)

Differential Diagnosis

- Primary open angle glaucoma • Chronic angle closure glaucoma • Inflammatory glaucoma • Pigmentary glaucoma • Bleeding disorder

Treatment

- Topical and/or oral hypotensive agents • Steroid drops • Cycloplegia • May need trabeculectomy or glaucoma drainage device if medical treatment fails • Hyphema may require anterior chamber washout if IOP persistently high despite therapy • Sickle cell patients with hyphema require close monitoring and lower threshold for anterior chamber washout • Avoid use of topical and/or oral carbonic anhydrase inhibitors in sickle cell patients with hyphema, because these drugs may contribute to metabolic acidosis and increased sickling

Prognosis

- Poor

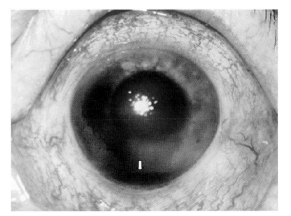

Fig. 6.26 Blood layering (arrow) in the anterior chamber (hyphema).

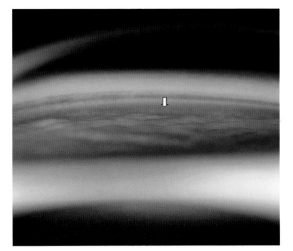

Fig. 6.27 Tear between the longitudinal and circular muscles of the ciliary body presenting as a widening (arrow) of the ciliary band (angle recession).

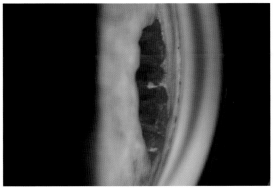

Fig. 6.28 A tear in the root of the iris (iridodialysis).

Uveitis–Glaucoma–Hyphema Syndrome

Key Facts

- Clinical triad found in some patients with anterior chamber lens implants, sulcus-fixated posterior chamber IOLs, or iris-clipped IOLs
- Increased incidence with anterior chamber lenses with rigid, closed loop haptics
- May present years after lens implantation

Mechanism

- Chronic rubbing from IOL haptics against iris, trabecular meshwork, and ciliary body

Clinical Findings

- Decreased vision
- Pain
- Photophobia
- Redness
- Recurrent hyphema
- Anterior chamber cell reaction (inflammatory and red blood cells)
- Pigment dispersion with iris transillumination defects (Fig. 6.29)
- Corneal edema
- High IOP

Ancillary Testing

- See *Primary open angle glaucoma* (p. 68)
- Ultrasound biomicroscopy
- Macular evaluation optical coherence tomography

Differential Diagnosis

- Trauma
- Inflammatory glaucoma
- Infection
- Neovascular glaucoma
- Coagulation disorders

Treatment

- Topical hypotensive agents
- Topical steroid drops
- Cycloplegia
- Lens exchange
- Vitrectomy may be needed if the vitreous is in the anterior chamber or adherent to the posterior iris

Prognosis

- Good if diagnosed early; however, diagnosis is often made late in disease course, with poor outcomes

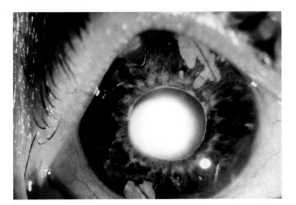

Fig. 6.29 Iris transillumination defects in a sulcus-fixated lens.

After Penetrating Keratoplasty

Key Facts

- Leading cause of blindness following corneal transplant
- Late glaucoma secondary to chronic angle closure with peripheral anterior synechiae formation
- Early elevated pressure secondary to inflammation, retained Healon, hyphema, angle closure, trauma, or angle compression due to over-tightening of sutures or small donor size
- Occurs in up to 31% in early postoperative phase and in 35% with long-term follow-up
- Increased risk in patients with history of glaucoma and aphakia
- Reduced incidence when donor corneal button is 0.5 mm larger than donor bed

Clinical Findings

- Corneal graft edema
- Corneal haze
- Pain
- Redness
- Decreased vision
- Peripheral anterior synechiae
- Excessively tight corneal transplant sutures
- Excessively large cornea donor graft may predispose to peripheral synechiae (Fig. 6.30)

Ancillary Testing

- Pneumotonometry is the most accurate way to measure IOP in patients with significant irregular astigmatism and corneal edema
- Pachymetry
- Visual field and imaging to test for optic nerve damage
- See *Primary open angle glaucoma* (p. 68)

Differential Diagnosis

- Primary open angle glaucoma
- Steroid response glaucoma
- Inflammatory glaucoma
- Neovascular glaucoma

Treatment

- Topical hypotensive agents
- Trabeculectomy successful in 69–91%
- Trabeculectomy results in corneal transplant graft failure in up to 18%
- Glaucoma drainage devices successful in up to 80% but frequently lead to graft failure
- Trans-scleral cyclophotocoagulation is successful in up to 80% but also leads to frequent graft failure

Prognosis

- Survival of graft is major factor in limiting visual function

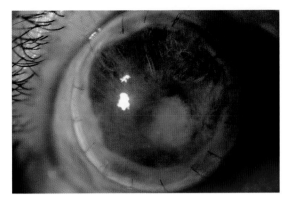

Fig. 6.30 Large cornea donor graft.

Hypotony Maculopathy

Key Facts

- Hypotony defined as IOP ≤5 mmHg but will vary based on central corneal thickness
- Maculopathy manifests with decreased and distorted visual acuity
- Increased incidence after trabeculectomy with antifibrotics (mitomycin-C and 5-fluorouracil)
- Increased risk in young male myopes
- Hypotony occurs in up to 30% of patients after use of antifibrotics during trabeculectomy
- Maculopathy occurs in approximately 10% of patients with hypotony

Mechanism

- Wound or bleb leak
- Over-filtration through sclerostomy site
- Cyclodialysis cleft
- Aqueous hyposecretion (possibly from mitomycin-C exposure)

Clinical Findings

- Decreased vision • Shallow anterior chamber • Iris and/or lens cornea touch • Anterior chamber cell reaction • Anterior and/or posterior synechiae formation • Corneal edema • Cataract formation • Choroidal folds (Fig. 6.31) • Macular edema • Optic nerve head swelling • Choroidal effusions

Ancillary Testing

- Dilated fundus examination
- B-scan ultrasonography may show choroidal effusions
- Optical coherence tomography to evaluate macula
- Ultrasound biomicroscopy may show cyclodialysis cleft
- Fluorescein angiography shows choroidal folds (Fig. 6.32)

Differential Diagnosis

- Bleb over-filtration • Aqueous hyposecretion • Wound leak • Retinal detachment • Choroidal detachment • Uveitis • Phthisis

Treatment

- Identify and manage underlying cause
- **Post-trabeculectomy:** most often will require surgical revision
- **Wound or bleb leak:** bandage contact lens, antibiotics, possibly aqueous suppressants, may require surgical correction
- **Over-filtering bleb:** autologous blood injection, laser to conjunctiva
- **Cyclodialysis:** close cleft

Prognosis

- Chance of full visual recovery decreases with increased duration of hypotony maculopathy

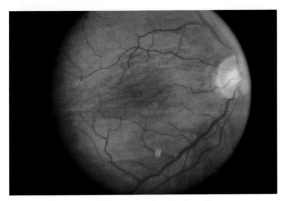

Fig. 6.31 Choroidal folds secondary to hypotony.

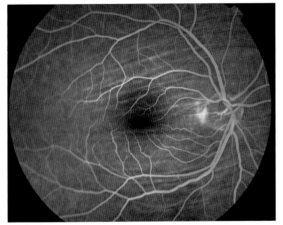

Fig. 6.32 Fluorescein angiography showing choroidal folds.

Section 7
Closed Angle Glaucoma

Acute Angle Closure Glaucoma

Key Facts

- Frequent cause for emergency room ophthalmic consultation
- Females more affected than males
- Higher rate in Asian and Inuit people
- Increased risk with hyperopia
- Increased rate with age, presumably due to increase in lens–iris contact related to lens thickness and cataract formation
- 5% of population over age 60 has occludable angles (0.5% of whom develop angle closure)
- Fellow eye has up to 80% chance of developing closure within 10 years

Mechanism

- Pupillary block causing bowing of iris forward and subsequent obstruction of trabecular meshwork

Clinical Findings

- Pain • Decreased vision • Redness • Photophobia • Shallow anterior chamber (Fig. 7.1) • Cloudy cornea (Fig. 7.2) • Haloes in vision • Peripheral anterior synechiae • Glaukomflecken (anterior subcapsular lens opacity due to lens epithelial cell necrosis) • Iris bombe (Fig. 7.3) • Mid-dilated pupil • Nausea and vomiting

Ancillary Testing

- Gonioscopy • Ultrasound biomicroscopy • Pachymetry • Possible need for endothelial cell count

Differential Diagnosis

- Inflammatory glaucoma • Neovascular glaucoma • Malignant glaucoma • Posner–Schlossmann syndrome • Phacomorphic glaucoma • Iridocorneal endothelial syndrome

Treatment

- Topical ophthalmic hypotensive agents
- Acetazolamide or methazolamide (oral)
- Oral glycerin
- Mannitol (intravenous)
- Laser peripheral iridectomy
- Consider prophylactic treatment of other eye if angle appears occludable
- Treat subacute and chronic form with laser peripheral iridectomy and hypotensive agent as needed
- Laser gonioplasty to break synechiae

Prognosis

- Poor if untreated and good to fair with treatment, depending on promptness of intervention

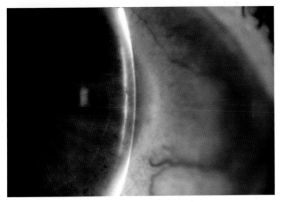

Fig. 7.1 Shallow peripheral anterior chamber.

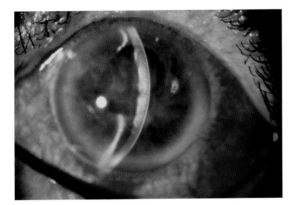

Fig. 7.2 Cloudy cornea with ciliary injection.

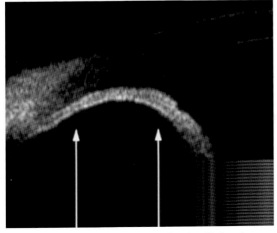

Fig. 7.3 Ultrasound biomicroscopy showing iris bombe (arrows).

Subacute Angle Closure Glaucoma

Key Facts

- Subacute or intermittent form presents with history of pain, decreased vision, and haloes but normal or mildly elevated IOP
- Examination shows narrow angle and few peripheral anterior synechiae

Mechanism

- Pupillary block causing bowing of iris forward and subsequent obstruction of trabecular meshwork

Clinical Findings

- Decreased vision
- Photophobia
- Haloes in vision
- Shallow anterior chamber
- Cornea usually clear
- Peripheral anterior synechiae
- Increased cup : disc ratio
- Glaukomflecken (anterior subcapsular lens opacity due to lens epithelial cell necrosis) caused by previous episodes of angle closure
- IOP usually normal or high normal at presentation

Ancillary Testing

- Gonioscopy
- Ultrasound biomicroscopy
- Pachymetry
- Possible need for endothelial cell count

Differential Diagnosis

- Inflammatory glaucoma
- Neovascular glaucoma
- Malignant glaucoma
- Posner–Schlossmann syndrome
- Phacomorphic glaucoma
- Iridocorneal endothelial syndrome

Treatment

- Topical ophthalmic hypotensive agents
- Laser peripheral iridectomy
- Consider prophylactic treatment of other eye if angle appears occludable
- Laser gonioplasty to break synechiae

Chronic Angle Closure Glaucoma

Key Facts

- Chronic form presents with few symptoms despite high pressure and diffuse peripheral anterior synechiae and narrow angle

Mechanism

- Peripheral anterior synechiae progressively occlude angle

Clinical Findings

- Decreased vision
- Shallow anterior chamber
- Clear cornea
- Diffuse peripheral anterior synechiae
- Glaukomflecken (anterior subcapsular lens opacity due to lens epithelial cell necrosis) as sign of previous acute angle closure
- Iris bombe may be present
- Nausea and vomiting with high IOP (IOP may be high normal or normal at presentation)

Ancillary Testing

- Gonioscopy
- Ultrasound biomicroscopy
- Pachymetry
- Possible need for endothelial cell count

Differential Diagnosis

- Inflammatory glaucoma
- Neovascular glaucoma
- Malignant glaucoma
- Posner–Schlossmann syndrome
- Phacomorphic glaucoma
- Iridocorneal endothelial syndrome

Treatment

- Topical ophthalmic hypotensive agents
- Laser peripheral iridectomy
- Consider prophylactic treatment of other eye if angle appears occludable
- Laser gonioplasty to break synechiae
- Many patients require trabeculectomy or glaucoma drainage device implantation

Narrow Angle Glaucoma: Nanophthalmos and Microphthalmos

Key Facts

- **Nanophthalmos:**
  - Axial length under 20 mm but otherwise normal eye
  - Small cornea
  - Lens large in relation to eye volume
  - Thick sclera with altered collagen architecture
  - Linked to MFRP gene
- Microphthalmos
  - Small deformed eye
  - Increased incidence of cataracts
  - Unilateral or bilateral
  - Association with CHARGE (coloboma, heart defects, choanal atresia, retarded development, genital and ear anomalies)
  - Usually autosomal recessive

Clinical Findings

- Small eye
- Small cornea (Fig. 7.4)
- Shallow anterior chamber (Fig. 7.5)
- Uveal effusion
- Hyperopia (extreme)

Ancillary Testing

- A scan to measure axial length
- B scan for uveal effusions
- Ultrasound biomicroscopy to evaluate anterior chamber architecture

Differential Diagnosis

- Microcornea
- Angle closure glaucoma
- Congenital glaucoma

Treatment

- Topical hypotensive agents
- Avoid miotics, which may decrease drainage angle width
- Laser peripheral iridectomy
- Incisional surgery
- Increased risk of choroidal effusion

Prognosis

- Glaucoma in the setting of nanophthalmos and microphthalmos difficult to treat and dependent on early diagnosis

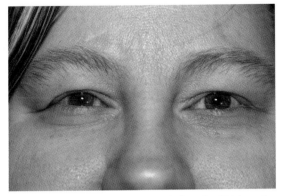

Fig. 7.4 Asymmetry between corneal diameter (right smaller than left).

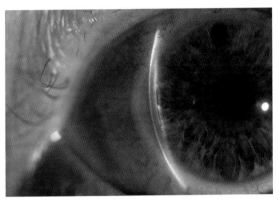

Fig. 7.5 Narrow angle in eye with nanophthalmos.

Plateau Iris

Key Facts

- Plateau iris configuration represents a narrow angle on gonioscopy with flat iris plane
- Plateau iris syndrome present when narrow angle (and possible acute closure) seen despite patent iridectomy
- Increased prevalence in young myopes
- Patients tend to be younger than population that has primary angle closure attacks

Mechanism

- Anterior position of ciliary processes pushes peripheral iris forward, occluding trabecular meshwork (Fig. 7.6)
- Anterior insertion of iris root

Clinical Findings

- Asymptomatic unless acute closure develops
- Pain
- Redness
- Decreased vision
- Closed angle with flat iris plane (no iris bombe as with pupillary block)
- Narrowing at drainage angle with sharp drop-off at peripheral iris
- Double-hump sign (Fig. 7.7) represents elevation of iris due to the lens, with more peripheral elevation caused by ciliary process indentation

Ancillary Testing

- Gonioscopy
- Ultrasound biomicroscopy

Differential Diagnosis

- Pupillary block
- Chronic angle closure
- Phacomorphic glaucoma
- Inflammatory glaucoma
- Malignant glaucoma
- Pseudoplateau iris configuration due to ciliary body tumor or cyst

Treatment

- Topical hypotensive agents
- Peripheral iridotomy if not done already
- Laser iridoplasty for plateau iris syndrome

Prognosis

- Good

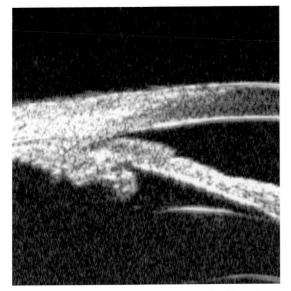

Fig. 7.6 Ultrasound biomicroscopy showing flat iris with loss of ciliary sulcus due to anterior position of ciliary process.

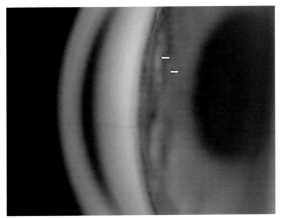

Fig. 7.7 Double-hump sign (arrows).

Phacomorphic Glaucoma

Key Facts

- The lens pushes the iris forward, causing pupillary block and closing the drainage angle
- Occurs with or without pupillary block
- Linked to advanced cataract (Fig. 7.8), traumatic cataract, and microspherophakia
- No sex predilection
- More common in hyperopic eyes with shallow anterior chamber

Clinical Findings

- Pain
- Redness
- Anterior chamber cell reaction
- Corneal edema
- Decreased vision
- Haloes in vision

Ancillary Testing

- Ultrasound biomicroscopy
- B-scan ultrasonography

Differential Diagnosis

- Primary angle closure glaucoma
- Plateau iris syndrome
- Inflammatory glaucoma
- Neovascular glaucoma
- Phacolytic glaucoma
- Lens particle glaucoma
- Presence of a phakic IOL

Treatment

- Topical hypotensive agents, possible need for oral agents in acute presentation
- Topical steroid drops
- Laser peripheral iridectomy
- Avoid miotics, which can cause anterior migration of lens–iris diaphragm
- Cataract extraction for definitive treatment

Prognosis

- Patients sometimes require continued treatment for IOP increases despite cataract extraction

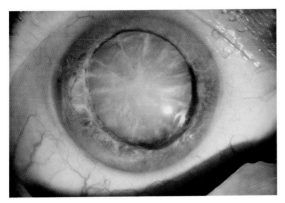

Fig. 7.8 Advanced cataract.

Neovascular Glaucoma

Key Facts

- Most commonly due to central retinal vein occlusion (CRVO) or proliferative diabetic retinopathy (PDR)
- Unilateral or bilateral
- Asymptomatic early in disease course
- Important to detect and treat early, because later stages have poor prognosis
- 30% of patients with neovascularization of the iris have diabetes
- 28% of patients with neovascularization of the iris have a CRVO

Mechanism

- Results from fibrovascular membrane growth over drainage angle
- Neovascular stimulus often due to retinal ischemia after vascular compromise (CRVO, PDR, central retinal artery occlusion, carotid disease, radiation, etc.)
- Vascular endothelial growth factor (VEGF) thought to be main mediator of neovascular formation

Clinical Findings

- Pain
- Redness
- Photophobia
- Decreased vision
- Non-radial fine branching vessels at pupil margin (rubeosis iridis; Fig. 7.9)
- A vessel crossing the scleral spur is abnormal (Fig. 7.10)
- **Stages:**
  - Stage 1: non-radial blood vessels along pupil margin and trabecular meshwork
  - Stage 2: stage 1 with high IOP
  - Stage 3: synechiae formation with closing of angle and diffuse iris neovascularization; can appear to have open angle, because once angle is zipped closed neovascularization in the angle is no longer visible

Ancillary Testing

- Fluorescein angiography
- Carotid ultrasound or angiography
- See *Primary open angle glaucoma* (p. 60)

Differential Diagnosis

- Primary open angle glaucoma
- Inflammatory glaucoma
- Neoplasia

Treatment

- Hypotensive drops
- Panretinal photocoagulation
- Glaucoma drainage device
- May need trans-scleral cyclophotocoagulation to control pressure
- Treat underlying disorder to reduce angiogenic drive
- Role of anti-VEGF medications being investigated

Prognosis

- Poor

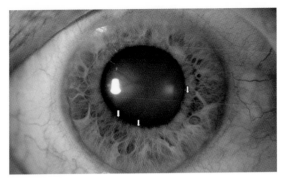

Fig. 7.9 Neovascularization of the iris.

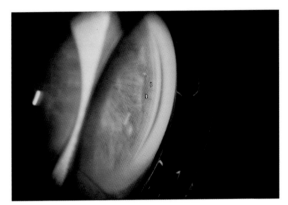

Fig. 7.10 Neovascularization of the angle.

Iridocorneal Endothelial Syndrome

Types

- Iris nevus syndrome (Cogan–Reese syndrome)
- Chandler syndrome
- Essential iris atrophy

Key Facts

- Involves corneal endothelium and associated iris abnormalities
- Unilateral
- Not heritable
- Increased risk in middle-aged women
- **Iris nevus syndrome:** corectopia and pigmented iris nodules resulting from contraction of proliferating endothelial cells
- **Chandler syndrome:** corneal changes with beaten bronze appearance to endothelium (Fig. 7.11)
- **Essential iris atrophy:** iris stromal loss with corectopia (Figs 7.12 and 7.13) and ectropion uvea

Mechanism

- Abnormal corneal endothelium proliferation and migration across trabecular meshwork and on to iris
- Endothelial cells appear metaplastic, with features resembling epithelial cells
- Cell migration across angle causes obstruction and elevated pressure, worsening with development of anterior synechiae (Fig. 7.14)
- Possible association with herpes virus infection

Clinical Findings

- Often asymptomatic
- Decreased vision
- Monocular diplopia (due to iris or pupil abnormalities)

Ancillary Testing

- See *Primary open angle glaucoma* (p. 60)

Differential Diagnosis

- Fuchs endothelial dystrophy • Trauma with iridodialysis • Inflammatory glaucoma • Posterior polymorphous dystrophy • Iris nevus, cyst, or tumor • Epithelial down-growth

Treatment

- Topical hypotensive agents if IOP elevated
- Corneal process may lead to penetrating keratoplasty

Prognosis

- Poor outcome when glaucoma present

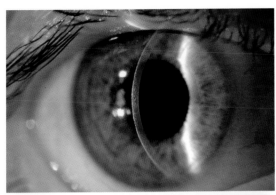

Fig. 7.11 Beaten bronze appearance to endothelium in Chandler syndrome.

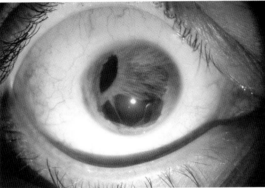

Fig. 7.12 Correctopia with iris atrophy.

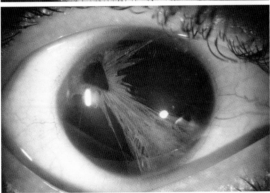

Fig. 7.13 Another example of correctopia with iris atrophy.

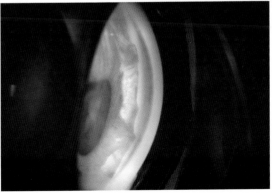

Fig. 7.14 Peripheral iris–corneal adhesions.

Aqueous Misdirection (Malignant Glaucoma)

Key Facts

- Occurs after or during incisional surgery or trauma
- May be induced by miotics even without surgery
- High rate after glaucoma filtration surgery
- Occurs in 0.6–4% of patients with angle closure glaucoma who undergo incisional surgery
- Cases have been reported after laser procedures and bleb needle revision

Mechanism

- Aqueous flow is misdirected into the vitreous cavity, with displacement of the vitreous forward toward the lens and iris
- The anterior chamber shallows, with resultant secondary angle closure and increased IOP

Clinical Findings

- Pain
- Redness
- Decreased vision
- Very high IOP
- Anteriorly displaced lens iris and ciliary body with shallow anterior chamber (Fig. 7.15)
- No iris bombe

Ancillary Testing

- Gonioscopy
- Ultrasound biomicroscopy
- B-scan ultrasonography

Differential Diagnosis

- Pupillary block glaucoma
- Choroidal effusion
- Suprachoroidal hemorrhage

Treatment

- Cycloplegia
- Aqueous suppressant drugs
- Miotics will worsen condition
- Peripheral iridotomy if angle closure suspected
- YAG laser to disrupt anterior hyaloid face
- Pars plana vitrectomy if condition does not resolve with other treatment

Prognosis

- Poor

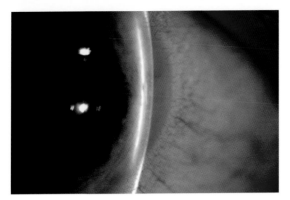

Fig. 7.15 Shallow anterior chamber with iris pushed against corneal endothelium.

Suprachoroidal Hemorrhage

Key Facts

- Devastating sequelae of incisional intraocular surgery or trauma
- Choroid and sclera normally in close apposition with no fluid in between
  - Hemorrhagic fluid fills this potential space after rupture of choroidal vessels
- No sex or race predilection
- Occurs with glaucoma surgery in 1.6% of cases
- **Increased risk with:**
  - advancing age • glaucoma • hypertension • tachycardia • arteriosclerosis
    - axial myopia • previous intraocular surgery • previous vitrectomy
      - aphakia

Mechanism

- Rupture of choroidal vessels with filling of potential suprachoroidal space and choroidal detachment

Clinical Findings

- Sudden excruciating pain with loss of vision
- Shallow or flat anterior chamber with or without lens–cornea touch
- Loss of red reflex (common intraoperative presentation)
- High IOP
- Domed brown elevation of retina (Fig. 7.16) with demarcation at site of vortex vein attachments
- May see touching of apposing choroidal elevations (kissing choroidals)
- May see vitreous hemorrhage and/or retinal detachment

Ancillary Testing

- B-scan ultrasonography shows dome-shaped elevations

Differential Diagnosis

- Retinal detachment
- Aqueous misdirection (malignant glaucoma)
- Serous choroidal detachment
- Pupillary block glaucoma
- Retrobulbar hemorrhage

Treatment

- Topical corticosteroids, cycloplegics, and hypotensive agents should be started immediately
- **Drainage of the choroidals advocated in cases of:**
  - kissing choroidals • high pressure uncontrolled with topical drops • lens cornea touch • persistent suprachoroidal hemorrhage despite treatment
- Timing of surgical drainage varies by surgeon preference and clinical picture
- Intraoperative presentation requires immediate intervention with sclerostomy placement to release the hemorrhage
  - Incisions are left open (not sutured closed) at the end of the procedure to facilitate further drainage

Prognosis

- Intraoperative suprachoroidal hemorrhages carry a worse prognosis because of loss of intraocular contents through surgical incision
- Loss of visual function in up to 80%

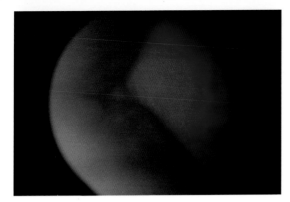

Fig. 7.16 Domed brown elevation of retina.

Aphakic and Pseudophakic Iris Bombe

Key Facts

- Frequency has decreased with modern cataract surgery
- Increased risk with anterior chamber and iris-fixated lenses
- Has been reported with posterior chamber lenses
- Decreased incidence with peripheral iridectomies and anterior vitrectomies in children

Mechanism

- **Aphakic iris bombe:** adherence between iris and anterior hyaloid face or vitreous with bulging forward of iris
- **Pseudophakic iris bombe:** adherence between iris and lens implant with bulging forward of iris

Clinical Findings

- May be asymptomatic
- Pain
- Photophobia
- Redness
- Corneal edema
- Iris bombe
- Peripheral anterior synechiae
- Synechiae to hyaloid face or lens implant

Ancillary Testing

- Gonioscopy
- Ultrasound biomicroscopy

Differential Diagnosis

- Malignant glaucoma
- Chronic angle closure
- Inflammatory glaucoma
- Neovascular glaucoma

Treatment

- Topical and/or oral hypotensive agents
- Topical steroid drops
- Cycloplegia to break or prevent synechiae
- Peripheral iridectomy

Prognosis

- Decreased incidence with modern surgery
- Good prognosis if discovered and treated early

Epithelial Down-growth

Key Facts

- Conjunctival epithelium grows into eye through penetrating wound or any incision that is incompetent
- Epithelium grows over corneal endothelium, trabecular meshwork, and iris
- Occurs in 0.09–0.12% of patients after cataract surgery
- Has been reported after clear cornea phacoemulsification
- May present decades after penetrating injury or intraocular surgery

Clinical Findings

- Thin gray translucent membrane growing over endothelium (Fig. 7.17) and iris (Fig. 7.18)
- Flattening of iris stroma
- Wound leak
- Peripheral anterior synechiae
- Pupillary block

Ancillary Testing

- Argon laser application to iris results in white burns in affected area (200-μm spot size at 300–500 mW)
- Gonioscopy shows peripheral anterior synechiae

Differential Diagnosis

- Inflammatory glaucoma
- Neovascular glaucoma
- Iridocorneal endothelial syndrome
- Acute or subacute angle closure glaucoma

Treatment

- Radical surgery to excise affected areas
- Glaucoma drainage devices have been effective in controlling IOP

Prognosis

- Poor because of high rate of recurrence and destruction of intraocular structures
- Results vary depending on degree of intraocular structure involvement

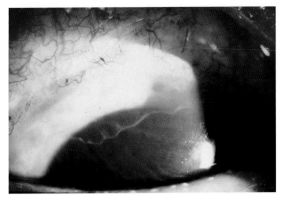

Fig. 7.17 Corneal haze with leading edge of epithelial cells on endothelial surface.

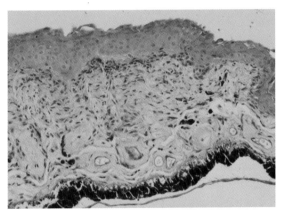

Fig. 7.18 Histologic section of iris, showing abnormal epithelial cell layer.

Section 8
Pediatric Glaucoma

Congenital and Infantile Glaucomas

Key Facts

- Congenital glaucoma present at birth
- Infantile glaucoma appears after
- Glaucoma not consistently associated with other ocular abnormalities
- Decreased aqueous outflow due to abnormal development of drainage angle
- Represents >20% of glaucoma in childhood
- 1/10 000 live births
- 80% present in first year of life
- Most cases sporadic
- 3 : 2 male : female ratio in the USA
- 65–80% bilateral

Clinical Findings

- Buphthalmos
- Increased corneal diameter (corneal diameter >12 mm in first year of life)
- Corneal edema (Fig. 8.1)
- Haab striae, which represent breaks in Descemet's membrane (Fig. 8.2)
- Blepharospasm
- Photophobia
- Epiphora
- Myopic shift

Ancillary Testing

- Dilated examination
- Gonioscopy
- Ultrasonography to record axial length
- Retinoscopy
- Pachymetry

Differential Diagnosis

- Lacrimal drainage system abnormality
- Megalocornea
- Birth trauma causing Descemet's membrane tears (Volk's striae)
- Corneal infections (acquired and congenital)
- Corneal dystrophies
- Peters syndrome

Treatment

- Goniotomy or trabeculotomy
- Older patients and those who fail initial surgeries may need trabeculectomy or glaucoma drainage devices in the future
- Hypotensive agents

Prognosis

- IOP controlled in 80% of patients with above treatments
- About 50% of patients have 20/50 vision or worse even with IOP control

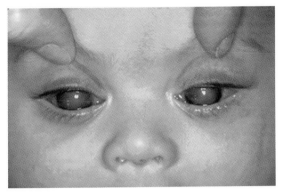

Fig. 8.1 Bilateral corneal edema in an infant with glaucoma.

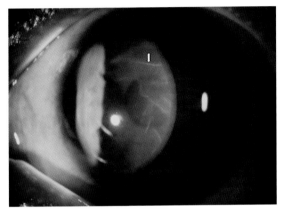

Fig. 8.2 Haab striae (arrow).

Axenfeld–Rieger Syndrome

Key Facts

- Bilateral congenital anterior dysgenesis of the anterior segment
- Autosomal dominant pattern of inheritance
- Linked to chromosomes 4q25, 6p25, and 13q14
- No sex predilection
- Posterior embryotoxon present in 8–15% of normal population
- Half of patients with Axenfeld–Rieger syndrome develop glaucoma

Clinical Findings

- Prominent anteriorly displaced Schwalbe's line termed *posterior embryotoxon* (Fig. 8.3)
- Peripheral iris strands (Fig. 8.4)
- Iris thinning and atrophy
- **Systemic abnormalities:** dental (Fig. 8.5), craniofacial, and skeletal (Fig. 8.6)

Ancillary Testing

- Goniosocopy shows peripheral anterior synechiae
- Systemic work-up

Differential Diagnosis

- Iridocorneal endothelial syndrome
- Peters anomaly
- Posterior polymorphous dystrophy
- Aniridia

Treatment

- May require goniotomy, trabeculotomy, and/or trabeculectomy
- Older patients treated with hypotensive drops and incisional surgery as needed
- Consultation of appropriate service for systemic abnormalities

Prognosis

- Success with trabeculectomy reported to be around 75% in older children and adults
- Prognosis of early onset glaucoma improves with early detection and intervention

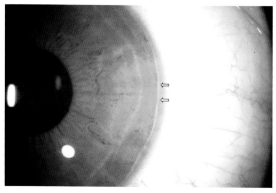

Fig. 8.3 Posterior embryotoxon (arrows).

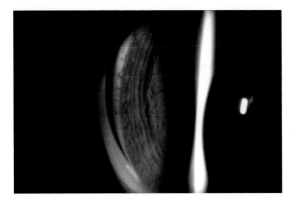

Fig. 8.4 Prominent peripheral iris processes.

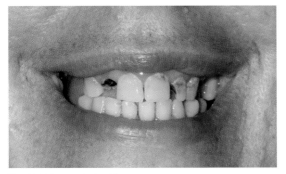

Fig. 8.5 Abnormal dentition.

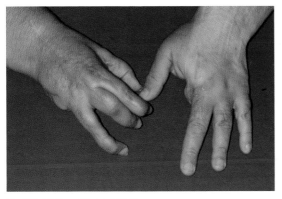

Fig. 8.6 Malformation of digits.

Peters Anomaly

Key Facts

- Rare anterior segment dysgenesis syndrome
- Caused by mutation in PAX6 gene
- Glaucoma due to angle dysgenesis
- Two types
  - Type 1: lens not adherent to cornea (80% bilateral)
  - Type 2: lens adherent to cornea (more likely to have systemic abnormalities)
- No known racial or sex predilection

Clinical Findings

- Central or paracentral corneal opacity (Fig. 8.7)
- Cataract with or without lens adhering to cornea
- Iris adhesions to cornea
- No vascularization of the cornea
- Microcornea
- Cornea plana
- Aniridia
- Reported associations with multiple systemic abnormalities

Ancillary Testing

- B-scan ultrasonography
- Ultrasound biomicroscopy
- MRI to rule out brain or spinal defects
- Abdominal ultrasound to rule out genitourinary abnormalities
- Cardiac echo

Differential Diagnosis

- Sclerocornea
- Posterior keratoconus
- Birth trauma
- Infectious keratitis
- Congenital hereditary endothelial dystrophy

Treatment

- Penetrating keratoplasty if indicated
- Cataract surgery
- Glaucoma drainage device
- Laser cyclophotocoagulation (trans-scleral or endoscopic)

Prognosis

- Visual potential usually 20/80 or worse after penetrating keratoplasty
- Early surgical intervention leads to better outcomes
- Visual potential worse when cataracts and glaucoma coexist

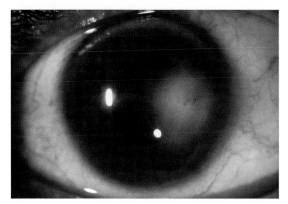

Fig. 8.7 Central corneal scar.

Aniridia

Key Facts

- Congenital absence of the iris
- Bilateral
- **Associated with:**
  - foveal hypoplasia • progressive peripheral corneal epitheliopathy • nystagmus • glaucoma
- Autosomal dominant inheritance
- PAX6 gene mutation on chromosome 11p13
- One-third of cases are sporadic
- Sporadic type associated with Wilms tumor

Clinical Findings

- Absent iris is common but iris morphology may be quite variable (Fig. 8.8)
- Patients have iris stump visible only on gonioscopy (Fig. 8.9)
- Peripheral corneal pannus and/or stem cell dysfunction advancing with age
- Foveal hypoplasia
- Nystagmus
- Hypoplasia of optic nerve
- May have cataracts

Ancillary Testing

- Systemic work-up including genetic consultation
- Rule out Wilms tumor

Differential Diagnosis

- Axenfeld–Rieger syndrome
- Sclerocornea
- Peters anomaly
- Iridocorneal endothelial syndrome
- Congenital nystagmus

Treatment

- Hypotensive drops for older patients
- Goniotomy and/or trabeculotomy for infants
- Trabeculectomy for older patients
- Tube shunt may be necessary for patients undergoing other anterior segment procedures, such as cataract surgery with artificial iris or limbus stem cell transplantation

Prognosis

- Glaucoma occurs in 50–75% of patients with aniridia
- Goniotomy may be a useful treatment for preventing the development of glaucoma in aniridia
- Trabeculotomy has high success rate for controlling IOP (up to 83% success)
- 68% of patients with chromosome 11 deletion develop Wilms tumor by age 3

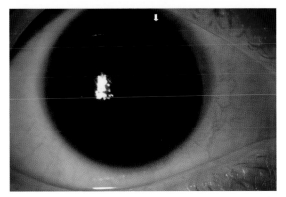

Fig. 8.8 Absent iris with visible lens equator (white arrow).

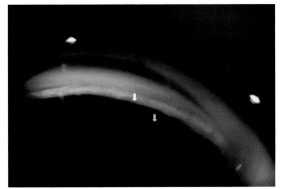

Fig. 8.9 Gonioscopy showing pupil remnant (white arrow) and visible ciliary processes (yellow arrow).

Neurofibromatosis

Key Facts

- Neurofibromatosis prevalence is 1/3000–5000 patients
- Glaucoma occurs in 1–2% of these patients
- Unilateral and present at birth
- Iris hamartomas (Lisch's nodules) increase with age (Fig. 8.10)
- Autosomal dominant
- Associated with chromosome 17
- May be due to developmental abnormalities of the anterior segment

Clinical Findings

- Café-au-lait spots
- Plexiform neurofibroma of upper eyelid (Fig. 8.11)
- Axillary freckles
- Iris hamartomas (Lisch's nodules)
- Ectropion uvea found more frequently in neurofibromatosis patients who have glaucoma (Fig. 8.11)

Ancillary Testing

- Similar to primary open angle glaucoma
- Gonioscopy
- Genetics consult

Differential Diagnosis

- Primary open angle glaucoma
- Congenital glaucoma
- Juvenile glaucoma

Treatment

- Hypotensive drops
- Trabeculotomy, goniotomy, and trabeculectomy

Prognosis

- 50% chance of glaucoma if eyelid plexiform neurofibroma present

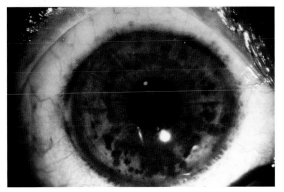

Fig. 8.10 Multiple iris Lisch's nodules.

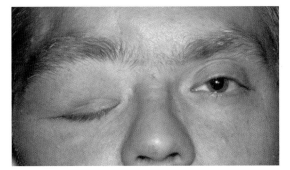

Fig. 8.11 Plexiform neurofibroma of right upper eyelid.

Posterior Lens Dislocation

Key Facts

- Displacement of lens into vitreous cavity
- **Occurs secondary to:**
  - trauma • intraoperative rupture of posterior lens capsule • pseudoexfoliation
    - inherited familial disorders (Marfan syndrome, Weill–Marchesani syndrome)
    - metabolic disorders (sulfite oxidase deficiency, homocystinuria)
- Immediate decrease in visual acuity
- Trauma and surgical complications are monocular
- Pseudoexfoliation, familial and metabolic disorders are bilateral

Clinical Findings

- Lens (either entire lens or pieces of lens material from surgery) in vitreous cavity
- Intraocular inflammation
- Elevated IOP from phacolytic glaucoma
- Vitreous hemorrhage from trauma or surgery
- Iridodonesis

Ancillary Testing

- Ultrasound if view to the retina is poor
- Evaluation for metabolic or familial disorders in conjunction with primary care physician

Differential Diagnosis

- Based on the metabolic or familial cause of the lens dislocation

Treatment

- Observation if no intraocular inflammation or elevated IOP from the dislocated lens
- Pars plana vitrectomy with lensectomy should be performed immediately after complicated cataract surgery or traumatic displacement of the lens if elevated IOP cannot be controlled with maximal medical therapy
- Surgical placement of an appropriate intraocular lens implant during vitrectomy surgery
- If no lens implant is performed, aphakic correction with contact lens may be used

Prognosis

- Good visual prognosis

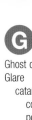

Index

electric shock, 42
inflammatory glaucoma, 66
Posner–Schlossman syndrome
(glaucomatocyclitic crisis), 80
Uveitis–glaucoma–hyphema syndrome,
92–93

Visual field defects, glaucoma
normal tension, 68
primary open angle, 60, 61

Vitrous hemorrhage
electric shock, 42
posterior lens dislocation, 136
suprachoroidal hemorrhage, 118
traumatic glaucoma, 90

Weill–Marchesani syndrome, 14, 20–21
posterior lens dislocation, 136
White cataract, 28, 29
Wilms tumor, 132